Nursing Research

For Churchill Livingstone:

Senior Commissioning Editor: Alex Mathieson/Jacqueline Curthoys
Project Manager: Ewan Halley
Project Development Editor: Valerie Dearing
Design Direction: Judith Wright

Nursing Research

Dissemination and Implementation

Edited by

Anne Mulhall BSc MSc PhD
Independent Training and Research Consultant, Woking, Surrey, UK

Andrée Le May BSc PhD RGN
Deputy Head of Department, Department of Health Studies, Brunel University, Uxbridge, UK

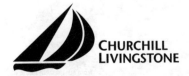

EDINBURGH LONDON NEW YORK PHILADELPHIA SAN FRANCISCO SYDNEY TORONTO 1999

CHURCHILL LIVINGSTONE
An imprint of Harcourt Brace and Company Limited

First published 1999

ISBN 0 443 05984 5

British Library of Cataloguing in Publication Data
A catalogue record for this book is available from the British Library.

Library of Congress Cataloging in Publication Data
A catalogue record for this book is available from the Library of Congress.

Medical knowledge is constantly changing. As new information becomes
available, changes in treatment, procedures, equipment and the use of
drugs become necessary. The editors / authors / contributors and the
publishers have, as far as it is possible, taken care to ensure that the
information given in this text is accurate and up to date. However, readers
are strongly advised to confirm that the information, especially with
regard to drug usage, complies with latest legislation and standards of
practice.

The
publisher's
policy is to use
**paper manufactured
from sustainable forests**

Printed & bound in India

Contents

Contributors

Nicky Cullum PhD RGN
Reader and Director, Centre for Evidence-Based Nursing, University of York, York, UK

Jacqueline Droogan MSc RGN
Research Fellow, NHS Centre for Reviews and Dissemination, University of York, York, UK

Beverley French RGN RMNH RNT MA
Lecturer, Faculty of Health, University of Central Lancashire, Preston, UK

Trudi James BSc MSc RGN DipHV
Research Fellow, Faculty of Health, South Bank University, London, UK

Anne Lacey BSc MSc RGN RNT
Research Fellow, School of Health and Related Research, University of Sheffield, Sheffield, UK

Jill Maben BA MSc RGN
Research Associate, Division of Nursing, King's College, University of London, London, UK

Pam Smith BNurs MSc PhD RGN DNCert HVCert RNT
Professor of Nursing, Faculty of Health, South Bank University, London, UK

Preface

There may be a gap between research and practice, but is there a gap between evidence and practice?

Although research-based practice has been promoted for the last 25 years within nursing, recent initiatives, such as the development of a Research and Development strategy for the National Health Service and the Culyer Report, have provided the organisational framework and resources through which this goal might be accomplished. Underwritten by a governmental policy seeking efficiency and effectiveness and the evidence-based movement in medicine, research-based nursing is now firmly on the professional and political agenda.

However, the problems of identifying research relevant to practice and ensuring its effective dissemination and implementation have been expressed internationally for a number of years – the so-called 'research–practice gap'. Moreover, hidden within this seemingly straightforward gap between the production of research and its application by practitioners are a number of complex factors. These relate in part to the ambiguity that research, and particularly 'scientific' research, has within nursing. For, although some are zealous in their enthusiasm for evidence-based nursing, others perceive it as too heavily weighted towards a biomedical model of disease and a governmental preoccupation with efficiency and effectiveness. Central to this debate is the question of what constitutes the activity of nursing and therefore what research, and indeed other types of evidence, are necessary to underpin it. Many nurses and the people in their care recognise the need for other evidence which arises from questions that cannot be conceptualised in scientific or economic terms.

The purpose of this book is not only to bring together the currently available information concerning the dissemination and implementation of research in nursing, but also to debate the issues raised above. All the authors have been directly involved with research in this area and each chapter provides both a synopsis of the current literature and insight into some of those studies most recently conducted in the UK. Our aim has been to gather together a diversity of viewpoints which at times may challenge the current status quo. Throughout, the intention has been to inform, yet provoke thought and debate.

The central role that 'evidence' is increasingly playing in the delivery of health care indicates that this book should have a broad appeal not only for practitioners, but also for managers and purchasers. Furthermore, although much of the research that is discussed and the debates that are raised are directly related to nursing, much of the information applies across disciplinary boundaries. Those working in the professions allied to medicine, and indeed doctors, may therefore also find the text useful.

1999

A.M.
A. Le M.

Introduction

Anne Mulhall   Andrée le May

RESEARCH AND THE HEALTH SERVICE

One of the underlying assumptions on which the National Health Service (NHS) is based is that the clinical professions within it consciously undertake and utilise research related to their practice (Kirk 1996). In order to sustain and develop this notion further, the 1990s have incurred frenetic activity by policy makers, professional groups, individual practitioners and service managers to ensure that care is based on appropriate evidence and provided within an evaluative culture. This prodigious effort has been associated with two factors:

1. The realisation that the practice of health care, regardless of the discipline of the professional delivering it, may have relied on unquestioned knowledge which, although it may have worked well, was at variance with the most up-to-date, critically appraised evidence.
2. The need to structure the knowledge that was available into an accessible format for use by practitioners working within a rapidly changing health care system in which time equates with money, and outcome often equates with increased throughput.

The goals for the 1990s and beyond are to: reemphasise the value of evidence-based practice (in which research plays a key role); encourage research that has a clear link to the practice arena; facilitate the dissemination and use of evidence; and provide practitioners with the skills to appraise evidence, implement it in practice and evaluate its effects on their care. In other words, to continue to bridge the gap between evidence and practice.

The history of research and development within the health service

To fully understand the rapid progress made during the 1990s towards evidence-based practice, we need to consider some of the central policies that have driven this agenda. Since 1989 there has been a central governmental push towards the active dissemination and implementation of evidence; indeed hardly a year has gone by without the publication of a policy document to guide us on our way (Box 1.1).

Box 1.1 Key publications in the development of an evidence-based culture in the NHS

1988	House of Lords Select Committee on Science and Technology: *Priorities in Medical Research*
1989a	Department of Health: *Priorities in Medical Research*
1989b	Department of Health: *Working for Patients*
1990	Richardson et al: *Taking Research Seriously*
1991	Department of Health: *Research for Health*
1991	Scottish Home and Health Department: *A Strategy for Nursing Research in Scotland*
1993a	Department of Health: *Research for Health* (second version)
1993b	Department of Health: *Report of the Task Force on the Strategy for Research in Nursing, Midwifery and Health Visiting*
1993c	Department of Health: *A Vision for the Future*
1994a	Department of Health: *Supporting Research and Development in the NHS* (Culyer Report)
1994b	Department of Health: *Testing the Vision*
1995a	Department of Health: *Methods to Promote the Implementation of Research Findings in the NHS*
1995b	Department of Health: *Consumers and Research in the NHS*
1996a	Department of Health: *Promoting Clinical Effectiveness*
1996b	Department of Health: *Research and Development: Towards an Evidence-based Health Service*
1997	Department of Health: *The New NHS: Modern. Dependable*

In the 1990s more emphasis than ever before has been placed on developing and articulating a coherent strategy related to:

- commissioning research
- funding research
- disseminating evidence from research and from other sources of knowledge to practitioners
- implementing evidence in practice.

This planned approach commenced with the government's response to the House of Lords' Select Committee on Science and Technology document, *Priorities in Medical Research* (Department of Health 1989a). This set out plans to improve the organisation and management of health research, thereby laying down the framework for Research and Development (R & D) over the following decade. The central objective of the strategy was to appoint a director of R & D who would advise the Executive on priorities for NHS research, and manage a programme of research in order to:

- meet identified needs
- focus on effectiveness and efficiency
- monitor support provided by the NHS for externally funded research
- ensure that research information was widely disseminated and used by practitioners and managers to improve patient care
- increase coordination between research funders.

These objectives have been systematically addressed since the appointment of the first Director of R & D in 1990 and articulated through a number of key policy initiatives (Box 1.1). As you can see, dissemination already formed a key component of the strategy and this was further strengthened through the recommendations that *Taking Research Seriously* (Richardson et al 1990) made to the government. Probably the first document to specifically focus on ways in which dissemination and implementation of research could be improved (Box 1.2), it made a considerable impact on the research community and laid down the foundations for much of the work that was to follow. As you read on you will see that many of these recommendations bore fruit.

Box 1.2 Recommendations focusing specifically on dissemination and implementation

1. To establish a strategic approach to dissemination
2. To provide support for dissemination to researchers
3. To provide more resources for dissemination
4. To consider the funding of research translators in order to meet the needs of multiple audiences
5. To consider mechanisms for dissemination
6. To study the ways in which research is used, how people find out about it and how utilisation could be enhanced
7. To identify research that is likely to be useful if funded
8. To commission literature searches and overviews
9. To encourage researchers to make findings 'salient to and understandable to those who will read them'

From Richardson et al (1990 p xiii)

The first major initiative came in the shape of the strategy *Research for Health* (Department of Health 1991), which has guided practice in this area ever since. The central tenet of this document was that R & D should become an integral part of health care and that all practitioners within the service would find it necessary (and natural) to rely on the results of research in their daily decision making. The launch of this strategy 'marked a shift in emphasis away from the NHS as a passive recipient of new technologies to a Service with a strong research infrastructure and competence capable of critically reviewing its own needs' (Department of Health 1993a p 4). The goal was to create a research-based 'service in which reliable and relevant information (was) available for decisions on policy, clinical practice and the management of services' (Department of Health 1993a p 4). To achieve this, close liaison was needed between all members of the research community, including:

- the director of R & D
- the regional directors of R & D

- the research providers
- the research funder
- the research users.

To further enhance the dissemination, and ultimately the implementation, of research, an information strategy was proposed which centred on the creation of three key structures, which are discussed more fully later in this chapter:

1. the National Register of Research (established by regional offices),
2. the Cochrane Centre, whose remit was the preparation, dissemination and maintenance of systematic reviews of randomised controlled trials of health care
3. the NHS Centre for Reviews and Dissemination, whose remit was to complement the work of the Cochrane Centre by commissioning reviews of research beyond the area of controlled trials and strategically disseminate up-to-date reviews into practice.

The next major objective was to focus on funding, and this gained recognition through the reporting of a task force chaired by Professor Anthony Culyer (Department of Health 1994a). This, in the main, tried to make sense of the myriad of funding arrangements that existed and to determine a coherent approach for the future. Key recommendations included that:

- a national forum to exchange information about the research strategies of those sponsoring or supporting R & D in the NHS be created
- there should be a single explicit funding stream for NHS R & D which would be financed by a levy on all health care providers
- the direct, indirect and service costs of R & D in NHS provider units, which were funded through income from patient care, were funded instead through the levy
- funding for research support should be available to primary and secondary care providers
- attention should be paid to the training and human resource issues related to R & D.

Four years on from the publication of this document, we have now reached a point when these key recommendations have been implemented, and you may be familiar with the extent of their success or failure from your involvement in the allocation of funds, the discussion of training issues or the impact of the levy on patient care.

Alongside the Culyer Report came a recognition that evidence would not be implemented into practice without considerable direction and effort: there were no magic formulae. Recognising this, funding for research to determine how best to disseminate evidence and consider its impact was made available (Department of Health 1995a). For many years we had been under the misapprehension that research findings diffused into practice effortlessly. However, gradually it was realised that this was not the case, and that effort needed to be concentrated on determining effective mechanisms for the dissemination and utilisation of evidence. It was clear that a strategy for research could not be merely a paper exercise: attention had to be focused in order to find out how best to move forward.

Of course the research strategy was not the only thing driving the agenda. The need to promote clinical effectiveness was (and is) its constant companion (Department of Health 1989b, 1996a, 1997). As a result of this movement towards clinical effectiveness came the recognition that evidence from randomised trials was not going to be available as a basis for all decisions. Indeed 'in (some) areas clinicians may legitimately draw upon analysis of expert opinion and past experience in the absence of such trials. The important point to remember is that all reliable information on effectiveness should clearly state the nature of its evidence-base' (Department of Health 1996a p 10).

Over the last 10 years, a myriad of governmental initiatives have been instrumental in refocusing our minds towards the evidence base for our practice, regardless of what that practice actually is. To do this: each individual practitioner is accountable for ensuring that his or her practice is based on up-to-date, critically appraised information; each researcher is accountable for taking steps to disseminate the findings of his or her work; and each manager is accountable for ensuring that practitioners have the facility to develop appropriate skills to ensure a real commitment to evidence-based practice. The time when care was based, unquestioningly, on ritual and tradition is long gone: we have entered an era when practitioners are expected to espouse the principles of lifelong learning, be provided with optimal access to information, and possess enhanced skills to use that information to achieve effective and efficient practice.

As the millennium approaches, there remains a firm commitment to an evidence-based health service (Department of Health 1996b, 1997), which is knowledge-driven and focuses on consistent access to services and the provision of quality care across the country. These objectives continue to be high on the new government's agenda and are articulated through their commitment to the formation of evidence-based national service frameworks and a new National Institute for Clinical Excellence designed to draw up new guidelines from the latest scientific evidence (Department of Health 1997).

Research traditions in nursing, midwifery and health visiting

As we have already seen, great attention has been focused, over the last decade, on policy which promotes evidence-based practice within an evaluative health care culture. Although Briggs (1972) is often held up as the forefather of research mindedness within nursing, midwifery and health visiting, it is clear that his recommendations are bearing more fruit in the 1990s than in the previous two decades. We are in the midst of an evidence-based practice revolution, in which an increased number of practitioners are actively undertaking research and utilising it in their practice.

The 1990s have heralded much change for the nursing professions. This has been facilitated by the movement of all of our education into the higher education sector: the realisation that although not all practitioners need to be researchers, they do need to be able to access, critically appraise and determine the clinical relevance and transferability of evidence to their practice; and the acknowledgement that unevaluated practice is unacceptable. Evidence-based practice has been put firmly on the agenda of all nurses, midwives and health visitors.

Despite this, nursing research has been described as 'fragmented, lacking a clear strategy and vision, and isolated from the wider body of research in the health arena' (Centre for Policy in Nursing Research 1997 p ii). Many of us would wholeheartedly agree and attribute this to a variety of factors (Box 1.3). However, it is fair to say that as a collection of disciplines which are seemingly 'new' to research, we are now beginning to formulate more coherent strategies for moving forward (Department of Health 1993b, 1993c) and determining priorities for research to drive the professions' agenda (English National Board for Nursing, Midwifery and Health Visiting 1995, Kitson et al 1997).

Box 1.3 Problems faced by nursing, midwifery and health visiting research

- Lack of history in research arena
- Distance between research and practice
- Minimal opportunities to link research careers to clinical practice
- Differing research traditions and power bases within health services research
- Limited educational opportunities to develop research skills
- Limited funding to develop research specific to nursing professions
- Lack of clear priorities for research specific to nursing professions
- Reliance on unquestioned traditional practices

One of the reasons often cited for the non-coherence of our approach has been the many research traditions in nursing, midwifery and health visiting. The complexity of the nursing professions' remit has led, naturally, to the use of various research designs which range from the experimental to the ethnographic (see Chapter 2). This breadth of approach has often, unfortunately, been seen as our downfall when compared to other health care research which more clearly focuses on the positivistic tradition of the natural sciences, but in reality, such eclecticism provides us with the advantage of being able to build our practice on a wide variety of evidence. However, whilst the rich collage of our knowledge, coupled with the range of research traditions available, best suits the complexity of our practice, the real issue remains of how to bridge the gap between the creation of evidence and its dissemination and implementation in practice. We hope that this book will contribute positively to this debate by providing both information and inspiration to readers.

DISSEMINATION AND IMPLEMENTATION: THE THEORY

As discussed above, current policy within the NHS R & D strategy strongly emphasises the need for individual health care professionals to base their practice on sound evidence. For nurses, midwives and health visitors, access to, and use of, reliable research-based evidence is implicit to the concept of autonomy promoted in the United Kingdom Central Council for Nursing, Midwifery and Health Visiting's Code of Professional Conduct (UKCC 1992). Similarly, *A Vision for the Future* (Department of Health 1993c) stresses the need for every nurse, midwife and health visitor to be able to recognise the role of research-based knowledge in the delivery of high-quality care. In addition, demands have been placed at a more organisational level on providers to indicate examples of where clinical practice has changed as a result of research findings. Tackling the issue from another angle, purchasers have also been exhorted to ensure that contracts for services state more specifically the extent of their research base.

From a purely theoretical standpoint, the drive to base more health care practice on rigorous evidence would seem both rational and relatively straightforward. If we have the evidence that a particular nursing intervention, say four-layer bandaging for the treatment of leg ulcers, works effectively then surely it is but a short step to the adoption of this method by all nurses who care for patients with this problem? Figure 1.1 depicts the thinking behind this sort of model. The evidence is produced, it is communicated to those who need to know, and they act swiftly on the information. However, even the most optimistic and starry-eyed member of the profession would question whether this would be the likely outcome. More probably you are sifting through a myriad of different reasons as to why, in practice, such an idealised scenario is highly unlikely to occur. In the first instance there is some reason to doubt how much of the evidence to underpin nursing actions currently exists. If there is no evidence, then by definition it cannot be used and we fail to move past first post in Figure 1.1. In other cases it is apparent that although information may exist, it has not been disseminated in a way appropriate to those making the decisions. For example, although the research evidence indicating that thrombolytic therapy following myocardial infarction is effective in reducing mortality was overwhelming by the early 1990s (Lau et al 1992), these findings were not

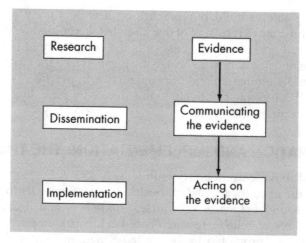

Figure 1.1 The process of dissemination and implementation of evidence in health care.

reflected in textbooks and review articles (Antman et al 1992). However, even when evidence is available and the relevant practitioners are aware of the optimal course of action on purely clinical grounds, other considerations (social, economic, cultural) may intervene to sway their decisions (Soumerai 1995). It is the very complexity of the model, depicted in such a deceptively simple way in Figure 1.1, which has been occupying the minds of those individuals and organisations who have begun more recently to address the issue of the dissemination and implementation of evidence in practice.

Since the principles underlying the dissemination and implementation of evidence for practice are, at least to some extent, generic, this field has attracted researchers and theorists from a wide range of health care professions. In consequence, terminology may vary. An essential starting point must therefore be a clarification of the ways in which the majority of authors in this book have defined certain words. The definitions below are, however, quite simplistic and each author may, in the relevant chapter, expand on them.

Defining dissemination and implementation

For the purposes of this book:

- *Dissemination* is defined as the communication of information to all potential 'customers'. These may include practitioners, clients/patients and their families, lay carers, educators, researchers, managers and policy makers.
- Evidence is *used* when it is accessed and evaluated with a view to

increasing knowledge and understanding. Use of research evidence usually involves searching the literature and critically appraising the articles found to be relevant to the subject at hand. Other types of evidence (see Chapter 3) may be accessed and evaluated in other ways.

• *Implementation* occurs when changes, based on the results of evidence, are made in practice. These activities rely not only on the availability of relevant knowledge, but more crucially on the critical evaluation of that knowledge. As we shall see later (Chapter 8 and 9), implementation is fraught with difficulties. It requires not only a means to translate knowledge from a variety of sources into the language and action of practice, but also the opportunity to elicit sustained change. Successful implementation depends on many factors. Some relate to characteristics of individual knowledge, ability and motivation, and others to wider politico-economic and organisational issues.

Four conditions are necessary for nursing practice to change as a result of research or other evidence:

• the availability of appropriate evidence
• the critical scrutiny of that evidence for rigour and applicability
• the conversion of that evidence into an applied form
• the acceptance of the evidence as legitimate, and its use as the basis for changes in managerial or clinical practice.

The history of dissemination and implementation

The dissemination and implementation of research evidence in health care practice has, over the last 10 years, gained an increasingly high profile within the UK. One of us (AM) well remembers how, when working in a Department of Health-funded research unit in the early 1990s, we progressively became aware that the implementation phase of research projects, and the time and resources that might be required for this, were being considered seriously by our funders. Some of the first indicators of this interest were expressed in such documents as *Taking Research Seriously: Means of Improving and Assessing the Use and Dissemination of Research* (Richardson et al 1990). People were realising that precious money was being spent on research (not just in nursing, but right across the health care disciplines) which subsequently never affected what happened either at an organisational level in terms of defining and delivering appropriate and effective services, or at the individual level of interactions between doctors, nurses and their clients. At the same time, as outlined above, the mechanisms for identifying, funding and providing research to meet the needs of the NHS rather than the needs of the Department of Health were undergoing a long, hard scrutiny. Integral to the new R & D strategy was the recognition that the dissemination and implementation of research was a research topic in its own right, and was furthermore a topic which for too long had been sadly neglected. A number of factors came together then to precipitate a new era of 'evidence-based practice' and 'clinical effectiveness' (more of these later). It became imperative that practice should be based on research, and where the evidence already existed, this indicated that structured efforts needed to be made to synthesise (or bring together) this evidence and present it in a way that was accessible to those who needed to use it: activities which lie at the core of dissemination and implementation.

Ironically, nursing, and particularly nursing in the USA, had already been exploring the issues of dissemination and implementation for the previous decade and a half. In the early 1980s, Hefferin et al (1982) noted that over 90% of nurse administrators agreed with the statement: 'it will be very important for nursing departments to be able to use the findings from clinical research studies which will be conducted in the coming years'. It is a revealing indication of the subordinate position of nursing within the health care hierarchy that this early work received little or no recognition, either then or now. Many papers (both theoretically and empirically based), models and innovative development ideas were put forward in the literature between 1975 and 1990. Some of this literature will be discussed here to give recognition to the importance of this work and to demonstrate the similarities that much of it has to some current initiatives. Examining this evidence provides us with three important lessons. Firstly, the need to thoroughly explore potentially rich sources of information across all the health care disciplines, and not to ignore work simply because it was conducted some time in the past or by other professionals. Secondly, it underlines the intricate partnership between knowledge and power: in this case the power of other groups such as doctors and general managers to recognise and legitimise particular knowledge that furthers their ends. Finally, it also demonstrates the abject failure of nursing to capitalise on an area where surely we could have indicated to the skeptics that we already had both the skills and the empirical research to offer this new and developing area. Perhaps failure is, however, the wrong word, for this example merely illustrates the strength of the socio-cultural forces that govern our actions and create the worlds in which we live. Those individuals, or groups of individuals, who hold power are able to perpetuate a particular set of circumstances and a 'set of mind', against which questions are framed and answers sought.

The purpose and importance of dissemination and implementation in nursing

It is impossible to deliver high-quality nursing care without the implementation of reliable evidence. In order to do this, evidence needs to be:

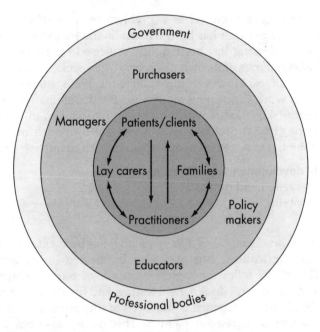

Figure 1.2   Evidence-based health care. Who is involved?

- available
- disseminated and understood
- relevant to practice
- incorporated into practice
- evaluated for its impact on practice.

The dissemination and implementation of evidence is a complex process which involves many key players (Fig. 1.2). However, it is a process which must be acknowledged and understood if a supportive basis on which to build practice relevant to the demands of health care consumers is to be developed. We hinted above that the sophisticated processes involved in dissemination and implementation, and the need to investigate them systematically, were recognised by nursing at least two decades ago. Addressing this, nurse researchers in the USA began to explore approaches used in other disciplines, and some of their work will be examined in the following section.

Models of research dissemination and implementation

The problem of dissemination and implementation is by no means confined to the health service. Other practice-based disciplines, such as social work and teaching, face similar dilemmas. Moreover, implementation has long been recognised as a problem in industrial research and development where much has been written on the subject by way of management texts. Nursing has been rightly criticised for its failure to look beyond the boundaries of its own discipline when seeking new knowledge or new perspectives. However, throughout the 1980s, nurses in the USA capitalised on work concerning models for the dissemination and utilisation of scientific knowledge which had been undertaken in the social sciences. Chrane (1985a) provides an overview of four such models which have the potential to be useful in applying research in nursing practice:

- research, development and diffusion
- social interaction and diffusion
- problem solving
- linkage.

The *research, development and diffusion* model has been extensively used in industry and agriculture, but may also be used to bring about social change. The model follows a logical sequence of pure research, applied research, conversion and design, field testing, and finally widespread diffusion. The innovator or scientist is the focus of this process, whilst the consumer is assumed to remain passive. This model assumes that if the innovation is properly developed, presented correctly and put forward at the right time, consumers will accept and use it. Criticisms raised include the model's focus on research and its inattention to the user (Havelock 1969).

The *social interaction and diffusion* model is perhaps most associated with the work of Rogers & Shoemaker (1971), and Stocking (1992) discusses it in an oft-quoted paper on promoting change in clinical care. The model describes the process involved when an innovation is communicated to the members of a social system (for example, the nurses working on one ward, or all of the health visitors in one practice). Rogers suggests that there are four factors which may influence whether 'innovations' (for our purposes these would be changes based on research or other evidence) are accepted and incorporated into practice. These factors largely revolve around the perceptions of those who are involved in bringing about the change or introduction of the innovation. The 'relative advantage' of a new practice, i.e. the extent to which it is perceived to improve on existing practice, is important. As Hardey (1994) points out, however, relative advantage is just that: relative. It is important, then, to explore how different individuals or groups who are involved in a change will be able to influence what occurs. Hardey cites the example of the routine induction of labour, which may have an advantage for some practitioners and institutions but is rejected by other health professionals and pregnant women. Rogers' model also highlights the importance that innovations are both 'compatible' with present practices and staff attitudes, and not so 'complex' as to be impossible for people to easily understand and implement. Finally, it should be possible to 'try out' innovations, perhaps in a demonstration area, and yet return to the former way of practice if necessary (trialability). Innovations that demonstrate high relative advantage and compatibility, lack complexity and have some degree of trialability are more likely to be adopted than changes that do not demonstrate these characteristics.

The rate of diffusion through the system is characterised by a predictable S curve of innovators who are willing to take risks, followed by early adopters or opinion leaders who must accept the change for it then to spread rapidly via the majority, until the whole process slows to a long late adopter or laggard phase. This model is backed up by a body of empirical research. However, it has been criticised for failing to appreciate the problems of effecting change within social systems (Havelock & Havelock 1973). Furthermore, its principal proponent, Rogers (1983), has revised his earlier thinking and accepted that adopters may not just be passive receptors and that innovations may arise at the operational level rather than purely from expert research sources.

The *problem solving* model (Lippitt et al 1958) incorporates a user-oriented approach to implementation. It encompasses a rational sequence of problem-solving activities including:

- the user realising and articulating a need which is transformed into a problem statement
- searching and retrieval to find a solution to the problem
- adapting the innovation to meet the needs of the user
- appraising the effectiveness with which the original need has been met.

The assumption here is that needs identified and 'solved' by the users themselves are more likely to be integrated and sustained in practice than innovations imposed by outside sources. Chrane (1985a) notes that although this model has great strengths, it does not specifically require the use of research evidence, and it may place excessive strain on the user organisation.

This leads naturally to the final *linkage* model put forward by Havelock & Havelock (1973) which attempts to use the best of the three previous models. The link is between the user system, for example a community health centre or a hospital trust (which has a system for identifying needs and its own internal problem solving system) and a resource system, which might be the nursing department of a university, that develops new knowledge and seeks user-relevant solutions to user problems. Needs and their potential solutions are transmitted from the user to the resource, who feeds back information on solution effectiveness and potential products or skills that may be required. The emphasis throughout is on a reciprocal partnership, where each system is able to simulate the problem-solving processes of the other. In this way, users learn to appreciate, say, how research knowledge and methods can be used, and the resourcers learn to understand the problems relevant to users. Moreover, the model is envisaged to extend beyond such partnerships to other resource systems to form a 'chain of knowledge utilisation' (Havelock & Havelock 1973).

The models described above were tested in a series of research utilisation projects undertaken in the USA between 1975 and 1985, including:

- the Nursing Child Assessment Satellite training projects (NCAST)
- the Western Interstate Commission for Higher Education (WICHE) Regional Program for Nursing Research Development
- the Conduct and Utilisation of Research in Nursing project (CURN).

Applying the models: early nursing research implementation projects

During 1976 to 1985, three NCAST projects were undertaken, all of which were based on Rogers' classic social interaction and diffusion model (see above). NCAST I tested the use of a communication satellite to disseminate research results, focusing on the reliability and validity of new assessment techniques related to child assessment. NCAST II used written materials, videotapes and satellite transmissions to facilitate participants' use of the new assessment techniques which they had become aware of through NCAST I. They thus practised assessments using videotapes of parent–child interactions and were also able to obtain inter-rater reliability on visits they made outside the classroom setting. The third project, Nursing Systems Toward Effective Parenting – Premature (NSTEP-P), aimed to teach public health nurses to use a protocol to follow up premature infants. Following a workshop on the content and use of the protocol, nurses returned to their practice settings and used the protocol for five cases. Help was provided during this time by telephone contact with the project staff and by a local mentor who had been trained in the use of protocols.

As part of the Regional Program for Nursing Research Development, the WICHE study was intended as a demonstration project through which models for overcoming the barriers to research implementation would be developed (Krueger et al 1978). Pairs of nurses from a variety of clinical settings attended a 3-day workshop where they learnt about research utilisation and the process of effecting change. Using the framework of the problem-solving model (see above), the nurses were helped to:

- identify a clinical problem
- locate the relevant research
- critique the research for rigour and applicability

- develop a plan for implementing the change to practice
- develop a plan to evaluate the effectiveness of the change.

The nurses then returned to their workplace for 5 months to try and implement the research-based change. A subsequent 2-day workshop explored their success in achieving this goal.

Initiated in 1975, the CURN project was conducted under the auspices of the Michigan Nurses' Association and used the linkage model (see above) as its theoretical basis. Using established criteria, the CURN project staff developed 10 nursing practice protocols which were based on a substantive body of rigorous research (CURN Project 1980–1983). Each protocol included:

- the clinical problem
- a summary of the research
- principles generated from the research
- how the innovation translated in terms of practice activity
- considerations for implementation and evaluation
- a bibliography
- the original research reports.

Teams of 6–8 nurses from different practice areas who would be responsible for implementing the protocol then attended 9 workshops over a period of 9 months. The workshops emphasised the use of research methods for practice and strategies for facilitating organisational change. The goal was to help practitioners to understand both how research methods could contribute to practice activities for example, by evaluating a change objectively, and how change could be effected with minimum disruption and maximum acceptance. The CURN project involved 34 nursing departments from various hospitals in Michigan, using both control and experimental sites. One year after the implementation of the project, experimental hospitals demonstrated a significantly higher level of research utilisation when compared with control sites (Horsley et al 1983).

These three projects demonstrate nurses utilising theoretical models and knowledge from other disciplines, in this case social science and management studies. Each project was based on a different model. The NCAST series used the social interaction and diffusion model which rests on the premise that knowledge moves through a social system in a predictable way which is determined by the ongoing social relationships within the system. It aimed to alert practitioners to new research and persuade them of its value. No efforts were made to directly change the practice settings in which the nurses worked. On the other hand, the WICHE project emphasised the involvement of the users in identifying problems themselves with subsequent facilitation to find the solutions to those problems. As Chrane (1985b) notes, this process is not tightly controlled and the user shapes the process as it moves forward. In contrast, the CURN project was based on a reciprocal relationship between the users of research and the knowledge-generating resource (the CURN project staff). The emphasis here was also on the use of research evidence, the use of research principles in nursing practice, and methods for changing the practice setting so that the innovation would be widely accepted. Several other models of utilisation have been put forward, including the Stetler/Marram model (Stetler 1994); the Iowa nursing project (Titler et al 1994); the Horn model (Goode & Bulechek 1992); and the Goode model (Goode et al 1987). Although these models do differ in their theoretical basis and indeed their application, White et al (1995) suggest that they all have important similarities: they are implicitly prescriptive; they indicate the steps and activities involved in utilisation; and they promote evaluation of findings for utility, feasibility and cost.

DISSEMINATION AND IMPLEMENTATION: THE PRACTICE

Earlier in this chapter, various theoretical models of research dissemination and implementation were explored and illustrated by the work that nurse researchers in the USA have undertaken in this field. In examining the different models, it is obvious that they are based on different ideas about how evidence might best be identified, evaluated, packaged, delivered and implemented, and importantly, who should be involved in such processes and at what stage. Is it up to practitioners to identify practice that needs changing? What part should professional bodies and government departments play? Where do the recipients of health care and their families fit in? Clearly the dissemination and implementation of research involves a number of groups of people such as nurses, doctors, patients, managers (who may be acting either independently or in unison) and also a number of organisational 'units' (ranging from small organisations such as community health centres to larger organisations such as hospital trusts and also the government). Figure 1.2 outlines some of those who may be involved and the potential forces, such as governmental policies, which may be acting on them.

Undoubtedly, the dissemination and implementation of evidence in clinical practice is not the straightforward exercise that we first envisaged in Figure 1.1, but is instead caught up in a complex system where individuals and organisations are acting against a backdrop of social structures, norms, policies and economic exigencies. Currently in the UK the NHS R & D Programme has precipitated a new surge of interest in this area, and a number of projects, initiatives and strategies have been set in train. It would be impossible to include all of them here, but the following three sections aim to provide some flavour of both the strategies involved and the different groups who are driving them.

Current strategies to promote dissemination and implementation

Initiatives taken by the government

The first two sections of this chapter describe the history of research and development within the health service in general, and nursing in particular. Within this overall strategy there are a number of specific initiatives which have been developed by the government to promote the dissemination and implementation of research. Three of the most important of these are the NHS Centre for Reviews and Dissemination (NHS CRD), the UK Cochrane Centre, and the National Research Register (NRR), all of which fall under the auspices of the NHS Information Systems Strategy (NHSISS).

The NHS CRD was established in 1994 and is located at the University of York. Its remit is to promote the use of research-based knowledge in health care by offering:

- systematic reviews of research on selected topics
- a database of good-quality published reviews
- a dissemination service.

The sibling organisation to the NHS CRD is the Cochrane Centre, which was established in 1992 to facilitate and coordinate the preparation and maintenance of systematic reviews of the effects of health care. These reviews usually utilise primary research studies which have used a randomised controlled design. The Cochrane Centre relies on the commitment of people who are willing to use their own time and resources to undertake and maintain reviews through one of the Centre's groups which focus on a particular clinical area such as pregnancy and childbirth, or wounds. However, to date few nurses have become involved in these activities (Dickson & Cullum 1996). These two initiatives, the NHS CRD and the Cochrane Centre, are described in detail in Chapter 6.

The NNR is a database of research and development projects currently taking place in, or of interest to, the NHS. Its objective is to supply more information about current research in the UK by providing:

- a tool to identify unwanted duplication of research projects
- a decision support for those commissioning research
- a basis for accounting for expenditure on research
- an input for research reviews.

To date (1997), the details from 6000 projects have been entered to include: the title of the research; the main research question; the lead researcher; the primary location of the research; and the methodology. It is anticipated that access to the NRR will be expanded shortly through the development of a CD-ROM version and the establishment of availability over the Internet and NHSnet.

The Nursing Research Initiative for Scotland (NRIS) is also undertaking systematic reviews of the literature with a particular focus on nursing. By May 1997 four reviews had been completed (palliative care services, 12-hour shifts, stress and quality of life among carers of the adult learning disabled, and stress and absence among nurses) (Hunt 1997).

Two important centres for the promotion of evidence-based practice have also been established through the NHS R & D Programme. The Centre for Evidence-Based Medicine was established in Oxford in 1995. It has three main objectives:

- to promote the teaching, learning, practice and evaluation of evidence-based medicine and health care
- to conduct applied, patient-based and methodological research to produce new knowledge required for the practice of evidence-based care
- to collaborate with scientists in the creation of a graduate programme to train researchers to perform randomised controlled trials and systematic reviews.

The Centre for Evidence-Based Nursing is based at the University of York. It is working with others to try and identify those areas of nursing where research and/or reviews of research are needed. Also underway is a major study exploring how nurses perceive and use evidence in decision making. Each of these centres produces a journal (*Evidence-Based Medicine* and *Evidence-Based Nursing*) which identifies high-quality, clinically relevant research papers and presents them as an abstract together with a commentary from a clinical expert in the relevant field. The aim of these journals is to serve practitioners by: bringing to their attention the findings of rigorous research; promoting the critical appraisal of research; and fostering implementation (Cullum 1996).

Within the NHS R & D initiative, the national programme on the evaluation of methods to promote the implementation of research is being managed from the NHS R & D Commissioning Unit based at NHS Executive North Thames. Twenty priority areas for this programme were established by a central R & D committee, and by February 1997 32 studies had been recommended for funding covering 13 of these areas. Updates on this programme are provided in the Research and Development Newsletter for North Thames (North Thames R & D Directorate, 40 Eastbourne Terrace, London W2 3QR).

Initiatives taken by regional NHS Executives

In addition to the national programme several regional NHS Executives have established networks and information facilities, organised training programmes, and funded R & D activities related to dissemination and implementation.

For example, North Thames R & D Directorate has set up the CHAIN (Contact, Help, Advice and Information Network) to enable all health care professionals who have an interest in implementation to identify and make appropriate connections with each other (Contact North Thames R & D Directorate or [http://www.nthames-health.tpmde.ac.uk/ntrl/chain.htm]). In late 1997 the Health Services Researchers' Network was integrated with CHAIN to provide a directory of health service researchers from a variety of disciplines who are able to furnish the NHS Executive, health authorities, trusts and academic departments with advice and expertise on particular health services research problems. Another initiative, the Aggressive Research Intelligence Facility (ARIF), centres on three departments at the University of Birmingham. ARIF was developed to provide a 'local' unit with responsibility for actively disseminating research information within one region. Uniquely, this unit has centred its activities on providing timely access to and advice on existing reviews of research to purchasers of health care. Each region also regularly produces a newsletter which outlines current programmes and alerts readers to future initiatives. These newsletters provide invaluable information and contact details for both local and national initiatives. For example, a recent newsletter from West Midlands region outlined commissioned research, the locally organised research scheme, regional research training fellowships, activities at Keele University, multicentre research ethics committees, and progress in national R & D initiatives. Newsletters are normally provided free of charge, or information and full text of reports may be obtained through the Internet. Another useful publication produced through the NHS Executive Anglia and Oxford is *Bandolier* (see also Chapters 6 and 9). This provides summaries and comments on recent research, book reviews and other information related to evidence-based health care. Currently much of its content focuses on medical issues, but it does attempt to cover concerns of interest to other disciplines.

Educational programmes developed through regions include research training fellowships which are open to most health care professionals, including nurses and scientific and managerial staff. Several regions also support training courses in the skills of critical appraisal, for example North Thames Research Appraisal Group (NTRAG) offers a series of workshops for health care personnel in the North Thames region, and a similar programme is run in Oxford and Anglia region: the Critical Appraisal Skills Programme (CASP) (see also Chapter 7). This type of workshop generally runs for 1 day and may focus on particular areas of care, for example primary care, topics such as guidelines, or particular research designs such as randomised controlled trials. To date these programmes have again had rather a medical flavour both in the examples chosen and the research designs discussed. However, the organisers are aware of a broader audience and are attempting to extend the scope of the programmes to include, for example, evaluation of qualitative research.

Alongside the national programme on the evaluation of methods to promote the implementation of research, regions have also funded their own programmes of research and development in this area. One which particularly focuses on nursing and midwifery issues is the South Thames Evidence Based Practice (STEP) project which is a collaborative venture between university departments of health care science, nursing and midwifery, and NHS trusts in South Thames region. Nine practice development posts have been established to implement evidence-based practice into a multiprofessional service setting and test its impact using a clinical audit framework. Areas of practice development include, amongst others, promotion of continence in primary care, increasing the uptake of breast feeding, family intervention in schizophrenia, and nutritional assessment and support of people with stroke in acute rehabilitation. This is but one example of the many projects funded through the NHS regional executives which have either been completed or are currently ongoing. Several of these, for example, the Assisting Clinical Effectiveness (ACE) Programme and the Scottish Intercollegiate Guidelines Network (SIGN) have focused on the production and/or implementation of guidelines for evidence-based practice.

Initiatives taken in Wales and Scotland

Many initiatives concerning the dissemination and implementation of research are currently being specifically developed in Wales and Scotland. The health services research (HSR) network in Scotland, as part of its overall remit to improve the quantity, quality and utility of HSR, will play a key role in the initiative to Get Research Applied to Scottish Practice (GRASP). This will encompass accessing and disseminating information from the Cochrane Collaboration, the NHSCRD and the NNR. The networks will also be involved in the diffusion of the CASP, which is aimed at health care professionals and managers in Scotland.

Initiatives taken by professional bodies and charities

In October 1996, the Royal College of Nursing (RCN) launched its Clinical Effectiveness Initiative with key aims to: develop the evidence base of nursing practice; provide information and education; and collaborate with other organisations to achieve more effective health care and contribute to the national agenda. Integral to the initiative is:

- the provision of a nursing and midwifery audit information service (free to nurses and midwives in the UK)
- the production and implementation of guidelines
- a series of educational programmes.

The information service includes a literature enquiry service, assistance with retrieval of information, help with audit activities, and access to a database of contacts who might be able to provide advice, knowledge and experience related to any particular topic of enquiry.

The RCN has also been involved in a joint initiative with the London School of Hygiene and Tropical Medicine to set up the Centre for Policy in Nursing Research (CPNR). Funded by the Nuffield Trust, the CPNR aims to provide a coordinated strategy for research in nursing, midwifery and health visiting, and to disseminate good practice (Centre for Policy in Nursing Research 1997). As a starting point it has been necessary to undertake a series of projects to establish the context in which nursing research is currently operating. Although the dissemination and implementation of research is often viewed at the level at which the research is to be applied, clearly contextual and wider policy issues may crucially affect these processes. Some of the projects that the CPNR will pursue will investigate these issues. For example, one project will explore the extent to which nursing research advice is utilised in central, regional and district level policy decision making; another the impact that particular pieces of research have had on research utilisation patterns; a third will review the constitutions and policies of funding bodies to examine perceptions of and interest in nursing issues. This wider and more policy-oriented perspective on dissemination and implementation of research may seem rather distant from the work of practitioners, but it is a critical component of the overall drive towards creating a balanced and equitable multidisciplinary approach to the utilisation of research in the health service.

Of course education is a crucial element in any drive towards more evidence-based health care. The development of the Project 2000 training for nurses (United Kingdom Central Council for Nursing, Midwifery and Health Visiting 1986) was a significant step towards this goal. The role of education and the implications of Project 2000 will not be further discussed here, as Chapter 7 addresses these issues, and explores in depth one of the studies commissioned by the English National Board for Nursing, Midwifery and Health Visiting (ENB) in this area. The ENB has also funded an Internet and CD-ROM project which provides information for educationalists, managers and practitioners in nursing, midwifery and health visiting [http://www.enb.org.uk]. Included are practice information in specialist areas, the ENB health care database, and educational research information.

Although many charities may support research on the implementation and dissemination of evidence in health care, one in particular, the Foundation of Nursing Studies (FoNS), has focused its efforts in this area. FoNS is involved in: funding projects which disseminate or implement proven research findings; partnering NHS trusts and other organisations in organising conferences; supporting networks and forums such as the

Professional and Practice Development Nurses' Forum; providing workshops on the utilisation of research and critical appraisal; and providing consultancy advice to NHS trusts and other organisations. (Further information may be obtained from the FoNS at 32, Buckingham Palace Road, London SW1W 0RE, or from the Internet [http://medweb.bham.ac.uk/nursing/fons.htm].)

This section on current strategies to assist the dissemination and implementation of research has focused on high-profile activities which have often received substantial funding. The range of examples offered above is by no means comprehensive, but it does provide an idea of the scope and depth of the undertakings currently underway. Clearly it is important for each of us to become familiar with those national and regional initiatives which may be useful, such as the NHSCRD or the work of the RCN with regard to clinical effectiveness.

What is the most effective way forward?

Several models of research utilisation were described earlier in this chapter. Strangely, whilst many of the current initiatives described in the section above address intrinsic elements of these models (for example, the NHSCRD and the Cochrane Centre can provide synthesised evidence for practice) little mention of this early work seems to be made, or indeed of the theoretical ideas that lie behind it. Whilst these models may be criticised as being too prescriptive and perhaps more relevant to the culture of health care in the USA where they were developed, having a clear framework for dissemination and implementation activities does have its advantages: not only by providing innovators with some concrete principles and activities to work by, but also in standardising strategies so that comparisons may be made across a number of sites and specialities to determine relative effectiveness.

However, the effectiveness of any one model or any strategy for change will depend on the context in which it is used. Thus a wise preliminary step in any dissemination or implementation activity is to carefully assess the current culture of research that exists in any setting. A first step is to gain some notion of how those practitioners, managers and educators who are being exhorted to increase evidence-based practice view this idea. There have been a number of studies recently in the UK which have explored the barriers to, and perhaps more importantly the opportunities of, evidence-based practice (see Chapters 4 and 8 for details). However, such studies only provide data on the perspective of individuals or groups of individuals to this problem. Whilst these perceptions are crucial, they must be complimented with other information which illuminates the contextual factors (such as the size and history of the health care setting, the skill mix of staff, the policy for staff development, etc.) which may encourage or impede a greater espousal of evidence-based practice. Such information is best gleaned from case history or ethnographic research which seeks to gain an insight into the 'whole picture'. This encompasses not only contextual issues as just described, but also an appreciation of where the particular topic or phenomenon, in this case evidence for practice, fits within the culture as a whole. What is its relative importance for both individuals and organisations compared with other activities and considerations?

Thus in moving forward, two considerations stand out. Firstly, more attention might be given to building on the early work from the USA, or at least in actively evaluating its worth for the UK setting. Secondly, more research, particularly of the type suggested above, is required to enable us to build up a more sophisticated picture of the cultures in which evidence-based practice is being promoted.

There is no doubt that the raised governmental awareness of the issue of clinical effectiveness has resulted in a number of valuable initiatives and organisations being set up, although sadly many practitioners remain in ignorance of the bulk of these activities. However, many developments are occurring at a more local level, often as collaborative ventures between NHS trusts and university departments. In Chapter 9, Jackie Solomon outlines one such partnership which evolved between Bolton Hospitals NHS Trust and Salford University to support the development of a nursing strategy for research and dissemination. Further contributors to the chapter describe other developments. Such initiatives are often reliant on the foresight and hard work of groups of professionals who strive, often with comparatively meagre resources, to advance evidence-based practice. Not only do they act as an excellent model of what can be achieved, but their grounding in the everyday contingencies of health care practice provides a welcome sense of reality. Such developments demonstrate what can be done by committed, flexible professionals working together at 'ground level'.

ABOUT THIS BOOK

At face value it could be suggested that this book is about the gap that exists between evidence, and in particular research evidence, and nursing, midwifery and health visiting practice. Moreover, the structure and content of the text is so arranged as to facilitate this approach. On one level then, each chapter may be read on its own or in conjunction with others to glean knowledge about the research–practice gap and the strategies which might help to bridge that gap. Thus Chapter 1 provides an account of research and development activities in the health service, and those initiatives, both past and present, which have been devised to ensure that practice is underwritten by such a research base. The other chapters develop in a logical sequence following the model of dissemination and implementation of research outlined in Figure 1.1. As portrayed in Figure 1.1, the model suggests that having identified the 'evidence' (and this is usually equated with research evidence), the job in hand is to 'communicate that evidence' effectively and efficiently to practitioners (dissemination) who will then 'act on the evidence' (implementation). Thus Section 1 examines the dissemination and use of research, and the chapters in Section 2 then discuss how implementation should occur through changes in practice.

However, as we recognised in Figure 1.2, the dissemination and implementation of evidence for practice is more complex, involving as it does a wide range of: individuals and groups, some of whom are acting in a professional capacity; health care organisations; society; and government bodies/policy.

Furthermore, it is clear that our thinking in this area has been less than rigorous. For example, it is assumed that there is a 'gap', that it needs filling, and that we know how, and with what it should be filled, and it must be said, who is largely responsible for the gap (the practitioner). Figure 1.3 attempts to expand on the dissemination/implementation model by posing a number of questions alongside the original steps. Currently we do not have the complete answer to all of these questions, and moreover, it is clear that some people and some organisations have in reality given these issues very little thought. For example, until recently

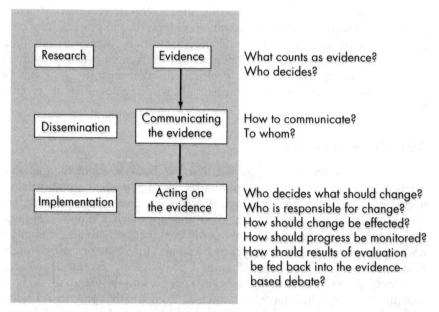

Figure 1.3 The process of dissemination and implementation of evidence in health care expanded.

there was an implicit assumption that the failure to underpin practice with evidence should be laid at the door of individual doctors, nurses or other health care professionals. That such individuals might be powerless to act, even if they had access to reliable evidence was not considered. The focus of the evidence-based movement on medical issues, 'scientific' research and the issues of effectiveness and efficiency has similarly squeezed aside the genuine concerns of other professions such as nursing, which do not share to the same extent the medical model of disease and care.

In their varying ways, the authors in this book have, alongside providing a certain component of basic information concerning the subject of their chapters, tried to delve more deeply into the more complex issues that the questions in Figure 1.3 raise. Thus Chapter 2 begins to raise queries about the whole premise underlying the model: that research-based practice as it is currently conceptualised is a 'good' thing, which given sufficient resources and enough application and energy will be both achievable and beneficial in terms of patient outcomes. In Chapter 3, the issue of knowledge, where it comes from, and what counts as evidence and who decides is faced headlong. These two chapters deal with these questions in a theoretical way, but in Chapter 9, Trudi James and Pam Smith illustrate these dilemmas through their case studies which explore the realities of attempting to implement research and development in everyday practice. In doing this, they too examine the nature of evidence, the philosophy and methods that underpin its production, and its relationship to practice.

Both of the next stages of the model in Figure 1.3 are affected by the attitudes which practitioners have to evidence. Obviously if practitioners are not aware of evidence then they cannot act on it, but their perceptions of the source of information (research, experience, significant others), the way it is communicated, who delivers the message and what it contains may crucially affect their acceptance and influence their subsequent actions. In Chapter 4, Anne Lacey discusses her own and others' work in this area and highlights the importance of taking a broad range of research approaches to investigating this area. Limiting research to more positivistic designs such as surveys using structured questionnaires or measurement scales will seriously impair any efforts to gain a more thorough understanding of why practitioners do or do not act. She also draws our attention to the similarities between nursing and other health care professions such as physiotherapy, occupational therapy and podiatry.

How to communicate and to whom? The poor communication of information is frequently cited as a major problem by different groups of nurses working in the health service (Foundation of Nursing Studies 1996). Information seldom seems to circulate in a productive way either at a micro level (say between individual nurses on a ward) or at a macro level through organisations. How often do you hear people say 'Well no one told me'? Chapter 5 provides a comprehensive review of the dissemination of research and suggests some innovative strategies which might enhance this process. However, we are cautioned to carefully examine the current strategies which are motivated by a vision that there are research resources that are under-utilised, which if tapped could benefit patient care. Such models ignore the role of dissemination in power relationships and the potential use of dissemination as a coercive strategy.

The dissemination of research and its use (conceived here as accessing and evaluating information) may blur together as activities. However, there is no doubt that for busy practitioners, both activities are problematic. Chapter 6 recognises the dilemma of health care practitioners who are faced with an overwhelming body of evidence of varying degrees of rigour through which they are expected to wade. It addresses these issues by describing how organisations such as the NHSCRD and the Cochrane Collaboration can both provide high-quality 'packages' of information and develop efficient, effective ways through which research may be best disseminated. These are vital resources for all the health care professions, and the nursing profession must ensure that it uses them to the full, participates in them, and engages in debate and communication as to what its particular needs from these organisations are.

Much of the debate surrounding the problems of dissemination and implementation revolves around the educational preparation of nurses. Using as her basis a major project commissioned by the ENB and her own doctoral work, Jill Maben in Chapter 7 focuses on the role of education in enhancing research awareness and subsequent dissemination and implementation. She notes the crucial importance of the environment in enabling newly qualified nurses to take forward the Project 2000 objectives of a questioning, research-aware practitioner. This raises some pertinent issues about who should decide what should change, and who is subsequently responsible for seeing those changes through. There are obvious dilemmas to placing such responsibilities with newly qualified staff.

Much has been written across a number of different literatures about change management. Chapter 8 explores some of these theories to ask the question of whether change can be managed. Juxtaposing the organisational development strategy with other approaches which find their underpinning in critical theory and action research, the author moves towards trying to identify an optimal approach to change in service organisations such as the NHS. In so doing, some of the questions about who decides what changes should occur, who is responsible for action, and how such strategies should proceed are addressed. Particular problems are identified with the concepts that underlie some models of change and how relevant they are for the NHS in general, and for nursing in particular. For the author the heart of the problem lies in the current dilemma in health care that much of the force for change and the evidence comes from the top, but the will must come from the bottom.

The final chapter of this book tackles the reality of making changes in practice. What really happens out there when people attempt to be innovative? Using their own research and case studies of four practice developments, Trudi James and Pam Smith draw together a convincing case for some of the theoretical observations made in previous chapters. In particular, they note how nurses make use of knowledge from a number of different sources. Thus the evidence from systematic reviews must be integrated with other forms of evidence that evolve from the disparate, disorderly complexity of elements that make up the socio-cultural world of nursing practice. Stemming from this is the need for nurses to have a firm grounding in research to enable them to be confident and knowledgeable enough to fully participate in creating a balanced multidisciplinary strategy for research. However much we might wish it were not so, support from those with power and influence is important, and other factors related to the environment in which research is applied must be fully considered in any implementation attempt. Fundamental to successful change is the need to make sure a mechanism exists for people to be heard and get involved, for them to have some ownership of the process of change. Central here is the building of relationships that promote communication and collaboration. The 'vision' of innovators needs to be a 'shared vision'.

Each contributor to this book has a particular perspective on the issues that they have discussed in their chapters. Sometimes this accords with the currently dominant views concerning the evidence–practice gap, and at other times authors have taken a radically different stance. We hope that this broad swathe of perspectives will provide readers with a variety of viewpoints and enable them to come to an informed yet balanced judgment as to their own position. Throughout, the intention has been to inform yet provoke thought and debate, and to topple presumptions and foster a critical stance in those who choose to read our efforts.

The dissemination and use of research

'Knowledge in a vacuum is fruitless, whereas knowledge used to enhance practice is of the utmost importance.'

2

A research culture?

Anne Mulhall

KEY POINTS

- Culture is a complex social phenomenon affected by individuals, groups and wider politico-economic forces
- It is difficult to define the parameters that accurately reflect the extent or nature of the research culture in nursing
- Nurses' positive attitude to research and a moderate level of research-based practice indicate that nursing is developing a culture of research. However, the research capital in nursing is still at a low level
- Two models of research culture emerge:
  - An eclectic model which adopts a variety of methodologies and techniques to tackle various questions
  - A more scientific/economic model which is emerging through the National Health Service Research and Development strategy
- Nursing research is socially constructed, i.e. individual researchers and the society in which they work will influence the questions asked, the methods used to answer the questions, and the way in which the answers are presented
- The economic/scientific discourse may silence important aspects of nursing which are intangible/subjective. Any legitimate research culture for nursing must recognise this and seek a more balanced perspective which encompasses research questions and research approaches which extend across the major paradigms

INTRODUCTION

In the preceding chapter we saw that an essential, if obvious, prerequisite for successful implementation is the existence of appropriate and rigorous research on which practice may be based. So although this book focuses particularly on the conditions and strategies which might favour effective dissemination and implementation, it is also important that we give some thought to both the substance and the nature of the information that is to be implemented, and to the culture into which it is to be 'delivered'.

The Briggs Report (1972) first formally suggested that nurses should base their practice on research. Since then, although it has been grossly under-funded in relationship to the number of nurses and the extent of their activities, research has been firmly on the policy agenda of both the government and the professional bodies (Department of Health 1993b, United Kingdom Central Council for Nursing, Midwifery and Health Visiting [UKCC] 1992). In addition, the importance of research has been underwritten by radical changes in pre-registration nurse education (Project 2000) and its integration into higher education, along with the increasing opportunities for nurses to gain postgraduate qualifications (see also Chapter 7). More recently there has been a growing concern not just about conducting research in nursing, but in ensuring its uptake in practice through improved dissemination and implementation (Department of Health 1993b, 1995a, Hunt 1996).

From a sociological perspective it is significant that nursing has felt the need to proclaim its espousal of research so clearly. Such a public articulation is an indicator both of the subordinate position of nursing in the health care arena, and the consequential desire of its leaders to elevate this status and gain the kudos of a 'profession'. In contrast, medicine historically has not needed to emphasise the research basis of its practice. Rather it has been assumed that, through its long and continuing research endeavour, medical practice would naturally be underpinned by rigorous empirical evidence. That this is not the case was acknowledged only recently in the wake of the evidence-based movement as discussed in Chapter 1. The issue of research-based practice, or rather the lack of it, is, then, firmly on both the nursing and medical agendas. Also uniting the health care professions are the consequences of the major reorganisations and changes of ideology that the National Health Service (NHS) has recently undergone. For a variety of reasons, which will be discussed in more detail later, these changes have thrust the movement for evidence-based health care to the forefront.

Nursing, like medicine, is faced then with the call to develop its research culture, and many individuals, professional organisations, educational institutions, and indeed the government itself, have responded to the call through various strategies, some of which are outlined in Chapter 1. All of these take for their premise the notion that research-based practice (as currently conceptualised) is a 'good' thing which, given sufficient resources and enough application and energy, will be both achievable and beneficial in terms of patient outcomes.

This chapter will explore these claims in greater depth, and together with some of the material in Chapter 3, will put forward a different set of arguments against which the move towards evidence-based health care in general, and evidence-based nursing in particular, might be viewed. The discussion will be framed around three questions:

- What is a research culture?

- Is there a culture of research in nursing?
- What sort of research culture does nursing need?

WHAT IS A RESEARCH CULTURE?

The word 'culture' seems to have seeped unnoticed into the language of the health service, and yet it is probable that many people if pressed would find it difficult to define. In anthropology, culture is defined as the system of shared ideas, rules and meanings which both inform us how to view the world and tell us how to act in it. Thus in our study of the research cultures of practitioners and managers (Foundation of Nursing Studies 1996, Le May et al 1997) we explored this concept within a framework which asked: What is research? What do practitioners feel about it? What do they think it could 'do' for them? What do they think they should do about it? Culture in terms of research was therefore not only about how nurses 'saw' research and reacted to it, but also how it impinged on their individual work practices and those of the organisation, and what might be achieved if research was more fully disseminated and implemented.

From this description it is easy to see that trying to change a culture is a complex task which needs to take into account many different factors which might attach both to individuals and to the wider structure of the organisations in which they work. For example, factors affecting the success with which individual nurses might base more of their practice on research include:

- their education: have they been taught the skills of critical appraisal?
- their ease of access to up-to-date research articles: is the library close at hand?
- the amount of time that they can allocate to such activities: are they overwhelmed by their clinical work?
- their professional position: are they able to suggest and/or make changes to practice?
- the 'atmosphere' of the unit/organisation where they work: is innovation encouraged and supported?

Some of the issues raised above which are related to the management of change will be explored in more depth in Chapter 8. For our purposes here it is important to grasp the idea that the ways and extent to which individual nurses will be able to act must be set against the wider constraints and opportunities afforded them in the workplace. Furthermore, arching over both the individual and the organisation is the wider socio-economic and political environment. As everyone who works in today's NHS knows, these represent powerful forces which can radically change the way in which health services are perceived, organised and delivered.

The last decade has witnessed a series of wide-ranging and fundamental changes to the NHS in the UK (Ranade 1994 provides an excellent account of these). These changes have affected both organisations and individual practitioners across the spectrum of health care settings. In particular, the institution of general management and the internal market has imposed controls on previously autonomous professionals whose activities had significant cost implications for the government (Traynor 1996). The major drive towards efficiency and effectiveness of clinical practice (NHS Executive 1996 p 11) is hardly coincidental. The government is looking to 'draw on the existing evidence of effectiveness to improve the quality of care our patients receive'. However, the issue of cost is also paramount 'In the longer term, we should invest in increasing the evidence-base on cost effectiveness' (NHS Executive 1996 p 11). Furthermore, although individual clinicians are being targeted by these initiatives, the major thrust is more likely to evolve through purchasers. 'Health Authorities and GP fund holders can use existing information to encourage NHS trusts to adopt more cost effective practices' (NHS Executive 1996 p 5). Thus decisions about care are increasingly to be grounded in a more comprehensive and rigorous appreciation of their effectiveness and cost effectiveness, and are at the same time moving further away from individual doctors and nurses.

Integral to the initiative for increasing the effectiveness of health care has been the development of the NHS Research and Development (R & D) strategy (Department of Health 1991). As explained in Chapter 1, the aim of this strategy is to create a knowledge-based health service in which clinical, managerial and policy decisions are based on sound information (Department of Health 1993a). A central research and development committee advises on priorities for R & D which thus far have closely followed several of the target areas identified in *The Health of the Nation* (Department of Health 1992), such as cardiovascular disease and stroke, mental health and learning disabilities, and cancer. However, the framework, tenor and language of the various committees, and the strategy documents produced have been criticised for concentrating on outcome to the detriment of process (Traynor and Rafferty 1997), and for being dominated by medicine and the scientific methods associated with a controlled quantitative approach (Scottish Office Home and Health Department 1991). These isolated protests aside, many of nursings' leaders have embraced research-based health care enthusiastically, perhaps in part to promote the professional standing of nursing, but also to protect its interests in an increasingly competitive workplace. Indeed some commentators have adopted an almost condemnatory stance, castigating nursing for concerning itself with qualitative research about, say, patients' and students' perceptions which 'do not necessarily reflect the needs of the NHS as a whole' (McLoughlin 1996 p 409). Instead, suggesting that nursing must 'participate in collaborative, multidisciplinary research, (to) acknowledge the need to learn from others and to acquire expertise, and credibility in the quantitative, outcome oriented methods which are required' (McLoughlin 1996 p 411).

In brief, nursings' formal response to the NHS R & D strategy has been depicted as reflecting 'the growing influence of managerialism, drives for efficiency in the Service as a whole and talk of client responsiveness' (Traynor & Rafferty 1997 p 30). In other words, either as a matter of professional survival and expediency, or because they actually perceive that the work and role of nursing within the multidisciplinary team is best served by such an approach, a large and influential sector of the profession has conceded to the model of research-based practice as perpetuated through the current NHS R & D strategy. The movement to research-based practice has been given further impetus through the introduction of evidence-based medicine and, more latterly, evidence-based nursing to the UK. Although the proponents of this approach to clinical decision making emphasise the part that different types of information, such as professional opinion, play (Sackett & Haynes 1995), 'evidence' has been widely translated by others as equating with the results of empirical research.

That the biomedical model of research (Box 2.1) may not provide all, or any, of the answers for nursing is raised by Lorentzon (1995). Hunter (unpublished conference proceedings, The role of consumers/users in evidence based health care, London, 1996) is more forceful in his analysis suggesting that evidence-based health care can be conceptualised as an integral component of the NHS reorganisations and represents the battle between corporate rationalism and professional monopolism, or to put it in simple terms, the struggle between governmental policy as enacted by general managers, and clinicians' power to make decisions about patient care. Evidence-based health care Hunter contends, 'strengthens dependence on the positivist tradition by reinforcing the belief that reality consists only of phenomena which can be quantified and measured'. Other means of understanding reality '... are rejected or displaced on the grounds of being unscientific'. In a similar vein, Lawler (1997) believes that the discourses of science and economics have shaped the way we think and talk about

---

Box 2.1 Biomedicine

The term 'biomedicine' is widely used, but remains rather ill defined. In general terms it refers to the predominant theory and practice of medicine in Euro-American societies. This is based on ideas of the body as a physical system and disease as a biological, rather than a social, category. Ill health in biomedical terms is largely based on demonstrating physical changes in the body's structure or function, each disease entity being recognisable by certain characteristics, and such diseases are then assumed to be universal in form and content. The ideas of natural science and in particular positivism (see Box 8.1) underly the theory and practice of biomedicine. The basic premises of biomedicine have been ascribed the following characteristics: scientific rationality; objectivity; and quantitative measurement.

nursing and yet have silenced important and central concerns to the discipline and its practice (see also Chapter 9).

It is time then to return to our original question: What is a research culture? This discussion has illustrated that culture is a complex phenomenon which may be affected by contingencies far beyond the immediate situations of nurses working in various parts of the NHS. At the current time, the culture of research in the NHS has been shaped by the exigencies of the health service reorganisations in general, and the particular influence that the NHS R & D strategy has wielded. This has led to a particular culture of research based largely on science and economic determinism. Later in this chapter we will consider whether such a culture of research is appropriate, or useful to nursing. However, before that we will explore how far nursing has adopted a research culture, and whether it offers any benefits either to nurses, nursing or patients.

IS THERE A CULTURE OF RESEARCH IN NURSING?

Two questions are relevant here:

- Firstly, to what extent has nursing adopted a culture of research?
- Secondly, what sort of culture has it adopted?

However, there are some considerable problems in trying to answer these questions. As indicated above, culture is a complex phenomenon, not easily captured by a distinct set of variables or measured by statistical means. So what will suffice as benchmarks to indicate the extent of the research culture in nursing, and the nature of that culture?

Returning to the definition of culture cited above, it is clear that culture has some influence on how people perceive things. So how nurses and those who work with nurses think and feel about research would be one indicator of the pervasiveness of a research culture. In addition, if culture also tells us how to act in the world, then it would be reasonable to assume that the extent to which practice is based on research should give us another indicator. Furthermore, nurses' perceptions of any gap between research and practice might also provide relevant information. Beyond the individual, 'research capital' might be measured by:

- the actual volume and quality of nursing research
- the extent of its funding base
- the percentage of nurses who undertake research degrees.

The nature of the culture is harder to capture, but nurses' expectations of what research might do for them certainly will give us some ideas about this. In addition, the range of methodologies that projects adopt and the questions that are asked would provide a flavour of the type of research culture that nursing is adopting. The rest of this section will summarise some of the research that has already been undertaken in the quest to provide this sort of information. Unfortunately, in some cases very little evidence exists upon which we might base our decision about the extent and nature of the culture of research in nursing.

The extent of the research culture

What do nurses feel about research?

A number of surveys have attempted to determine the factors that affect research utilisation in nursing, and in so doing have investigated nurses' attitudes to research. This work was pioneered in the USA where nursing has been much concerned with the issue of implementation for the last 25 years. Bostrom et al (1989), investigating the attitudes of 720 staff nurses from a teaching hospital using the Boothe Attitudes on Nursing Research Scale (Boothe 1981), reported that many nurses were interested in research. Similarly, Marsh & Brown (1992) confirmed Chenitz et al's (1986) finding that nurses held moderately positive attitudes to research, but also reported that attitude improved with increasing education and exposure to research activities. Registered nurses in other countries demonstrate similar attitudes; Ehrenfeld & Eckerling (1991), in a study of 166 nurses in Israel (approximately one-third of whom held degrees), reported that research activities were perceived as important.

In the UK a number of studies covering a broad spectrum of nurses confirm that research is held in a positive light. An early pilot study of F and G grade nurses working in two sites (a district general hospital and a high-profile teaching hospital) indicated that nurses had an overall positive attitude to research (Lacey 1994). This was confirmed in two large studies which took random samples, ensuring a more representative picture. The first investigated 398 nurses working in a variety of settings including hospitals, health clinics, colleges of health and psychiatric hospitals (Pearcey 1995) and the second surveyed 500 nurses selected nationally and drawn from all grades (Hicks 1995). Examining other sectors, Veeramah (1995) reported that over 90% of a sample of 118 mental health nurses agreed that the application of research-based knowledge was essential for practice, and Meah et al (1996) found that midwives considered research to be highly relevant to their practice.

Many of these studies used structured questionnaires asking for answers to such statements as 'I want to base my practice on research', and attitude scales. The limitation of this approach is that participants may respond with the correct, or expected, answer. The advantage lies in the large sample sizes and greater representativeness that such studies incorporate. However, it is important that these quantitative approaches are complemented by qualitative studies such as Bassett's (1994) phenomenological

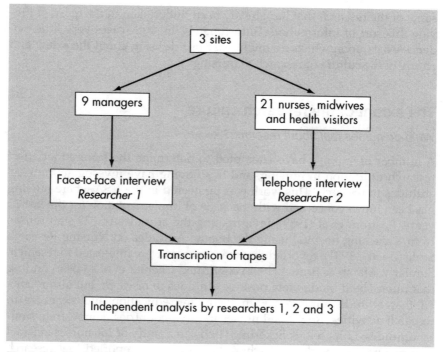

Figure 2.1 Design of study.

study of nurse teachers' attitudes to research, and also our own work with practitioners and managers (Le May et al 1998). Using semi-structured interviews we explored the culture of research of 21 nurses, midwives and health visitors and nine managers (chief executives, directors of nursing services and R & D nurses) from three health care sites across England. Figure 2.1 and Box 2.2 illustrate the design of this study, the interview prompts and the process of analysis.

Table 2.1 summarises practitioners' and managers' attitudes towards research. Practitioners revealed an intriguing paradox of fear/excitement, wariness/desire for involvement. In contrast, managers never expressed these 'emotive' elements, but rather noted more hard-headed strategic or planning issues such as how it was necessary to be cautious, research was a luxury, but they also recognised the importance of maintaining a positive stance. However, although these two groups held different views, it is clear that research had a high profile in the culture of both practitioners and managers.

Nevertheless, in appraising such studies it is important to examine carefully both the composition of the study group and the response rate. It would be reasonable to assume that those who do not respond to questionnaires or offers to be interviewed are perhaps less likely to view the subject

---

Box 2.2 Interview prompts and process of analysis

Interview prompts
Practitioners:
- Describe your feelings, experiences and reactions to the ideas of research and how it affects what you do every day
- In what ways does research guide you when working with patients?
- Have you experienced any barriers to developing research-based practice?

Managers:
- Tell me about the research and development in this trust
- What are the funding structures for R & D in this trust?
- Are there any particular issues which jump out for you, you think need to be changed, or get you excited or annoyed?

Process of analysis
1. Bracketing of researchers' experiences
2. Transcripts checked by participants
3. Independent review of transcripts by three researchers. Extraction of significant statements. Clustering in themes
4. Significant statements checked by participants
5. Consensus on significant statements and themes (credibility/reliability check)
6. Compilation of exhaustive descriptions by researchers 1 and 2 (interpreter triangulation)
7. Amalgamation of exhaustive descriptions for each site by researcher 1 Credibility check of these by researcher 3
8. Descriptions to participants to compare with their own experiences
9. Final version of exhaustive descriptions

Table 2.1 How do we perceive the world? Practitioners' and managers' attitudes to research

Practitioners	Managers
Site 1	
Worried and panicky	Cautious
Excited	Reinventing the wheel
Unsure about what is available	Associated with individuals
Want to be involved	
Site 2	
Must be nurse-led	A luxury
Must have practice focus	Sidelined
Alien/scary/phobic	Done by individuals
Trendy	The way forward for nursing
We do it/they may not	
Intriguing	
Site 3	
Sceptical	Proactive
It's new	Committed
Hard work	Nurses are leading the way
Done by others	Done by practitioners
Excited	

in question, i.e. research, positively. Our own study may have been biased in that only one-third of those approached agreed to be interviewed, and likewise some of the quantitative studies (Hicks 1995, Marsh & Brown 1992) had low response rates. However, the remainder achieved acceptable rates of over 60% and included samples representative of a wide range of clinical situations and educational backgrounds. It is reasonable to conclude therefore that both quantitative and qualitative studies indicate that general nurses, mental health nurses, midwives and health visitors view research in a positive way and regard it as important to base their practice on research evidence. How far do these perceptions, however, guide their practice? They see research as important, but does this translate into the way they act in the world?

How much practice is based on research?

Approximately 25% of nurses in two large studies carried out in the USA report using research to change practice (Bostrom & Suter 1993, Rizzuto et al 1994). In the UK, information is more limited. Armitage (1990) suggested that little research was being used in practice, but Lacey (1994) reported that about 50% of nurses used protocols based on research, and Veeramah (1995) cites 55% of nurses in mental health settings as using research 'to some extent'. Meanwhile, governmental figures (Department of Health 1994b) suggest that 86% of units have changed clinical practice as a result of research findings. Who should we believe? Clearly these discrepancies in estimates of research-based practice are a direct result of the variety of ways in which this attribute is being measured. Are we talking about all, some, or a few practices? How has compliance to a standard of research-based practice been measured and how was the standard derived? These are thorny issues which will require considerable effort and debate to resolve at both a theoretical and a practical level. Certainly a more universal application of relevant and useful clinical audit might provide some of this missing evidence. However, until there is some consensus on a definition of research-based practice, it is difficult to assess the extent to which nurses are acting on their positive image of research and using it to guide their actions. There is no doubt, however, that both researchers and practitioners talk about the gap between these two domains.

The research–practice gap

The entire rationale of this book rests on the assertion that there is a gap between research and practice. Research exists, but practitioners, be they doctors, nurses or other health professionals, fail to act on this evidence (Oxman 1994, Walsh & Ford 1989). Many theorists have discussed this gap and proffered reasons for it (Hicks & Hennessy 1997, Mulhall 1997, Rafferty et al 1996, Rolfe 1994), but what do practitioners think?

Most of the respondents in our study acknowledged that there was a gap between research and practice. Often this was related to the clinical area in which they worked: 'In some departments on the wards they are more aware and there is not a research practice gap there' , or in contrast, 'It was because we were very much isolated in theatres'. Various explanations for the gap were offered. Poor communication and dissemination were often cited, with practitioners remaining unaware of important research findings. However, there were other manifestations of the gap. Much research was considered as irrelevant to the questions that practitioners were raising; other studies lacked generalisability, and some findings had unrealistic resource implications. However, it was not only the research output that caused problems, but the researchers themselves. Researchers were seen as pursuing academic goals, not practice goals: 'Full time researchers may be working their own agenda and may not be dealing with issues pertinent to practice', and 'They did not ever get back to us to tell us what the results were, but we could read the paper in the magazine, it was up to us whether we read it or not'. Managers also envisaged researchers in a particular way: 'If you were to ask me to give you a picture of a researcher, then a nursing researcher is someone definitely not wearing a uniform, probably walking around with a great pile of books and papers, and somehow the patient is a bit off there'.

These responses give us some powerful clues to understanding why a gap exists between research and practice. Much nursing research in the UK is undertaken in establishments of higher education but, despite efforts to collaborate, the discipline-oriented university and the practice-oriented service continue to hold different values and beliefs. Those organisations involved in the purchase and provision of health services (such as hospital and community trusts and health authorities), and those involved in the education of nurses and the pursuit of research (such as universities, colleges of health and research units) will have different agendas (Mulhall 1995). Furthermore, individuals within these organisations will have their own particular goals. Academic researchers have some freedom to tackle particular research questions, the pursuit of which may or may not result in clear-cut results. In contrast, the exigencies of practice mean that nurses, midwives and health visitors must seek optimal and unambiguous answers to practical problems. It has been suggested, therefore, that there is a dichotomy between the attainment of consensual knowledge which typifies nursing as a profession, and the critical and inquiring position taken by academic knowledge (Chandler 1991). This gap will stultify attempts to increase the culture of research in nursing. However, it seems that recent governmental strategies, whilst they may be criticised for focusing on effectiveness as conceptualised within a biomedical model (see Box 2.1), have raised the profile of research within trusts (Department of Health 1994a). Moreover, there is evidence that some nurses at least have been able to capitalise on this to increase the culture of research both within their own professional groups and across other health care disciplines. Chapter 9 provides some innovative examples of nurses' work.

Research 'capital'

As noted above, further, more global, indicators of the existence of a research culture would include an inventory of research activity in nursing, its funding base, and the number of nurses obtaining research degrees. Fortunately, just such an exercise is being undertaken by the Centre for Policy in Nursing Research (CPNR) (see Chapter 1). Researchers there are undertaking a mapping exercise of research activity to collate information about project funding, the methodologies that projects have used, their geographical distribution, publications, and postdoctoral completions throughout the UK. Unfortunately, as nursing research becomes increasingly subsumed within health services research in general, it becomes more difficult to identify studies or activities that might be categorised in the domain of nursing. However, using the NHS National Research Register (see Chapter 1), the CPNR has determined an estimate of nurse-led projects in the NHS. Only a small proportion of projects (58–82) out of a total of 6413 projects registered were nurse-led. In addition, from information held by the Royal College of Nursing and the British Library, they have been able to map a steady increase in the number of completed PhD theses related to nursing between 1976 and 1993, with a levelling off since then (Rafferty & Traynor 1997). However, the absolute number is relatively small, standing at 226. With the total number of practitioners on the UKCC register for 1995 being 642 951, this represents a minute percentage of the total workforce.

The nature of the research culture in nursing

The CPNR mapping exercise, when complete, should also provide information concerning the types of methods and methodologies that are being used and the questions that are being asked. This will provide urgently needed data which will both define the culture of research in nursing more clearly and identify potential strategies for setting a national agenda. The nature of the research culture may also be captured by exploring what practitioners think nursing does, and could do, for them. Table 2.2 illustrates our finding related to this. Although participants had had difficulties in defining research, a strong theme emerged of research as the route to validated, standardised and evaluated practice. Research was construed positively by practitioners as a rational basis for practice and the enhancement

Table 2.2 How do we act in the world? What practitioners thought research does, or could do, for them

Practitioners	Managers
Site 1	
Improves care	Enhances trust's reputation
Justifies practice	Enhances trust's image
Justifies staffing	Attracts dynamic staff
Leads to ritualistic practice	
Would it change practice?	
Site 2	
Guides and improves care	Motivates staff
Solves problems	Gives staff confidence
Gives confidence	Gives staff autonomy
Gives the profession credibility	
Standardises care	
Site 3	
Tells us what to do/not to do	Raises trust's image
Validates practice	Raises nursings' profile
Standardises practice	Marks trust as innovative
Evaluates practice	
Improves care	
Gives credibility	
Develops practice	

of the profession. Some practitioners also indicated a notion of research as being fully integrated, almost second nature: 'Part of everything which we do'. Managers meanwhile projected research as a maker of images, a hallmark of quality and efficiency which could be linked to the corporate objectives of the trust.

In summary, although there are obvious gaps in the knowledge base, overall the studies reviewed in this section indicate that nursing has, or is fast developing, a culture of research. What is less clear is the nature of that culture. A certain dichotomy seems visible. The academic nursing journals portray the research culture in nursing as encompassing an extraordinary range of methodologies and methods and a variety of philosophical stances, ranging from positivism to critical theory. However, a reading of much governmental policy documentation and the thrust of newer journals would reveal a different emphasis, focusing on efficiency, effectiveness and cost considerations and, considering this subject matter, a not unreasonable affiliation to more quantitative methods and measurable outcomes. Although it may be stretching the data too far, it seems that the research culture of the participants in our study more closely matched this latter model. Given the mechanisms through which the NHS is funded and the policy directives to which it must comply, this is unsurprising. Furthermore, with the implementation of the recommendations from the Culyer Report (Department of Health 1994a) (see Chapter 1) moving research more within the structure of the NHS, this trend is likely to intensify. In addition, the identification of an activity called nursing research is fast disappearing from official terminology as it becomes subsumed into health services research. All this will have the effect of moving research in nursing closer towards the models of economic determinism and health technology which are enshrined in the NHS R & D programme. Our question now must therefore be: Is this the culture of research that nursing, and the recipients of nursing care, need?

WHAT SORT OF RESEARCH CULTURE DOES NURSING NEED?

Before attempting to answer this question, it is important to consolidate some of the arguments that have emerged from the discussions above. Running through all these is the idea that nursing research is socially constructed. But what is meant by this?

The social construction of research

The idea that research might be a construct, or if you like, a product, of the society in which it exists was initiated by the work of Thomas Kuhn (1970). Kuhn's arguments are summarised by saying 'that data or observations are theory laden (that is the scientist only sees data in terms of their relevance for theory); that the theories are paradigm laden (explanations are grounded in world views); and that paradigms are culture laden (world views including ideas about human nature, vary historically and across cultures)' (Nielsen 1990 p 13). Thus scientific theory may be socially and historically grounded, and scientists' values and judgments may fuse with the more 'objective' criteria by which competing paradigms are judged. These ideas spawned a spate of work by sociologists such as Latour & Woolgar (1979) who first described how laboratory science was not actually an objective, value-free endeavour, but was instead socially constructed. Thus scientists, and the context in which they are working, influence the types of questions that are tackled, the way in which the questions are approached and the final framing of the results or scientific facts. More recently in nursing, Porter (1993) has criticised the assumption that the attainment of objective knowledge through the setting aside of a researcher's values and interests is possible. Subjective, value-laden choices are made throughout the process of research by individuals who are working at a particular time and in a particular context (Ratcliffe & Gonzalez-del-Ville 1988). These newer ideas therefore both challenge the conceptual basis of science and promulgate the view that knowledge is socially constructed, and as such cannot be disentangled from the perspectives of researchers themselves.

The social construction of research in nursing

Building on the arguments above, it is quite possible to discern a number of characteristics which might illustrate how nursing research has been social-ly constructed. The introduction to this chapter discussed how research has been taken up by nursing in an effort to professionalise its activities. Used in this way, research is an instrument for advancement of a social group: nurses. Thus it has become a symbol of professionalisation, and as our study of practitioners and managers indicated, a hallmark for good prac-tice, quality, efficiency and innovation. Research could be said to have assumed a persona that goes beyond its role in providing the evidence upon which good practice should be based, it is something more than this, it has been constructed as an ideology. I would also suggest that hegemonic processes are at work within nursing research. Hegemonic processes occur when subordinated populations participate in cultural constructions (or ideas) that contribute to their continuing subordination. Research has become a culture in which both practitioners and researchers collude. Perhaps as a result of nursing's long struggle for academic recognition, research has always held mystical qualities as a higher-order pursuit only to be tackled by those who have finally made the grade to the top of the profession (often, unfortunately, leaving the practice arena as they do so). In this way research acts as an occupational strategy which sets boundaries around the professional territory of researchers (Mulhall 1997) and excludes those who don't do or cannot understand research.

This may all seem a far cry from trying to determine the sort of research culture by which nursing might best be served. However, it is necessary to appreciate that research is not simply a value-free exercise conducted to benefit patients and clients. It may act in all sorts of other roles and serve a range of different interests. Accordingly, the nature of our research activi-ties, the methods that we use and the questions that we tackle are affected by these 'social' contingencies. This presents a dilemma, however, for if everyone has a particular self-serving agenda, how should we choose which culture of research to foster in nursing?

Which culture?

Dingwall & MacIntosh (1978) point out the obvious attractions that the research traditions of an established profession, such as medicine, would have for a young discipline, such as nursing. This would therefore account in part for the attachment of early nurse researchers to the methodologies and practices of natural science. Almost as a backlash to this 'hard science' approach, qualitative researchers emerged who contested that the social world could not be investigated and understood in this way. But these researchers may in their own way have added to the drive for professionalisation by emphasising that nursing was underpinned by a unique knowledge base different from that of medicine. More recently, the pressure of the NHS reorganisations and the subsequent attention to efficiency and effectiveness has rekindled an espousal of more quantitative methodologies which can provide measurable outcomes. Clearly research is being driven by more than an altruistic desire for knowledge and best practice.

Seeking the best format for our research culture demands that we acknowledge those factors which impinge on every aspect of this domain: infrastructure; funding levels; 'acceptable' methodologies; 'appropriate' questions; and answers that are deemed as useful. From this perspective, the trend towards subsuming nursing research within health services research is worrying. Not because there is anything wrong with health services research, or that it cannot offer nursing some very valuable answers to its questions, but because the key stakeholders in this domain are not nurses. Why should this matter? This matters because knowledge is inextricably linked to power (Foucault 1980) and thus those in a position of power are able to delineate what counts as legitimate knowledge, and the ways in which such knowledge may be expressed (see also Chapter 3). Historically, medical knowledge has been assigned unquestioned authority. Moreover, the mechanisms through which dominant voices come to exercise their control remain disguised or ignored. The problem with the evidence-based movement is that it risks handing power to those with the wherewithal to produce the type of evidence currently in favour, i.e. the evidence which emerges from large randomised trials (Healy 1997). If, as Rafferty & Traynor (1997) imply, nursing research has suffered a profession-based disadvantage resulting in an underdeveloped research culture, then we are not in a position, either now or in the future, to produce this particular type of evidence, and perforce gain the power to shape what counts as legitimate knowledge. Or to put it in simple terms, if we cannot afford the fare to get on the train then we will be unable to direct where the train might go, or where it might stop on the way.

The current focus on evidence from randomised trials is problematic for a profession which has taken caring as central to its activities. For although much of the technical aspect of caring requires data from trials of effectiveness, much else subsumed within this concept cannot be explored using the methods of natural science. This has led for calls to adopt a methodological pluralism whereby health care research combines a variety of approaches to produce both qualitative and quantitative evidence (Avis & Robinson 1996). But until those in power acknowledge the social conditions of knowledge production, and therefore their role in shaping knowledge, it is likely that such calls will remain unheeded.

Lawler (1997) discusses this dilemma in terms of how nursing is being 'invited' to formalise its knowing and researching of the body. She suggests that knowledge of the body in nursing has been regulated and controlled by dominant economic and scientific discourses. Nursing, she contends, 'is concerned with things, like feelings and emotions of the body, which the academy has difficulty in accommodating' (Lawler 1997 p 35). Yet the imperatives of economic determinism have forced nurses to formalise their knowledge in a way which is more meaningful to managers and economists than to practitioners. Lawler (1997 p 48) continues to explain that although nursing requires research focused on biological events, because it is concerned with living people this must be accompanied by data derived through the social sciences lest 'we lose the focus on being human and embodied'. Finally she argues that knowledge must be derived from the practice of nursing – being and doing nursing. However, her caveat is that although nursing may borrow methodologies it must remain alert to the limitations of what it borrows or has thrust upon it 'so that we reflect nursing and not nursing-through-the-world-of-others' (Lawler 1997 p 49).

Lawler's emphasis on the importance of knowledge derived through the business of practising nursing echoes the work of Schon, whose seminal work on the reflective practitioner highlights the deep seated nature of the problems of professional knowledge, which will be more thoroughly explored in Chapter 3. Schon (1983 p 42) remarks how 'In the varied topography of professional practice, there is a high, hard ground where practitioners can make effective use of research based theory and technique, and there is the swampy lowland where situations are confusing "messes" incapable of technical solution. The difficulty is that the problems of the high ground... are often relatively unimportant to clients or to the larger society, while in the swamp are the problems of greatest human concern'.

This quotation seems particularly appropriate to our attempts to define the sort of research culture which nursing and its clients might best be served by, for it raises three crucial questions that encapsulate the contents of this chapter and which I will leave you to consider:

- Is nursing all 'swamp'?
- Have we got any research about the 'swamp'?
- Will the current structures under which research knowledge is produced facilitate the production of 'swamp' knowledge?

The next chapter will begin to unravel some of these questions by exploring the different types and sources of knowledge in nursing.

3

Knowledge for dissemination and implementation

Andrée le May

KEY POINTS

What is knowledge?

- Nurses, midwives and health visitors use many types of knowledge
- Knowledge, per se, may be difficult to define

Why do we need knowledge?

- Knowledge supports practice in a variety of ways
- Different types of knowledge are associated with different currencies
- Knowledge is being repackaged to encourage us to use it

How is knowledge articulated and disseminated?

- Practitioners use formal (e.g. through publication, conferences) and informal (e.g. reporting, mentoring) routes
- Much knowledge is passed on through the oral tradition

How is knowledge implemented?

- Practitioners implement knowledge invisibly and visibly
- Implementation is complex and requires specific skills
- Knowledge for nursing, midwifery and health visiting practice is dynamic

INTRODUCTION

It is not my intention, in this chapter, to enter into a long and complicated debate on the nature of knowledge; many have done this before, and interested readers will find several eloquent and thought-provoking discourses on this (for example, Robinson & Vaughan 1992). My concern here is more pragmatic: to raise some questions which will help us consider the impact of knowledge on the process of dissemination and implementation of evidence. The following questions structure this chapter:

- What is knowledge?
- Why do we need knowledge?
- How is knowledge articulated and disseminated?
- How is knowledge implemented?

In raising these questions I do not intend to furnish readers with definitive answers, as that is an impossibility; my intention is to draw you into the debate and help you to come to your own conclusions. These will impact, in turn, on a wide range of nursing, midwifery and health visiting practice through patient/client care, education, research or management.

WHAT IS KNOWLEDGE?

On the face of it, this seems simple to answer; after all, we must know what knowledge is, since we all value it greatly, search for it as if it was a holy grail and when we find people who we recognise as knowledgeable, we treat them with respect and hold them in high esteem. Knowledge would therefore seem to have considerable societal and professional currency. But when one asks practitioners what knowledge is, one is often met with uncertainty – the seemingly simple is surprisingly complex to define. The dictionary definition appears straightforward enough, stating that knowledge is 'what a person knows: the facts, information, skills and understanding that one has gained, especially through learning or experience' (Longman 1991 p 581). So it must be the relationship between practice and knowledge that adds difficulty. This is probably because knowledge for practice is so all-encompassing. The complexity of practice, with its different foci, may make it hard to identify exactly where our knowledge for practice originates. This hesitancy in isolating and defining knowledge may affect the ways in which we:

- generate knowledge
- articulate and disseminate knowledge
- search for knowledge
- use knowledge
- evaluate the impact of knowledge on practice.

This is further complicated by the variety of specialism(s) within which we practice in nursing, midwifery and health visiting, and the diversity of the other professions with whom we deliver our practice. Knowledge may mean different things to different people.

To a certain extent, the assumption that we use different 'knowledges' in our practice is supported in the nursing literature since a variety of types of knowledge are proposed (for examples see Carper 1978, Hagell 1989, Meerabeau 1995). The classification of these varying and complementary types of knowledge appears to centre on the origin of that knowledge; they may be classified as:

- theoretical
- empirical
- practical

Box 3.1   Types of knowledge

- *Theoretical knowledge* is frequently linked to knowledge which is not generated through research or practice, but through a process of logical thought. In some instances you may find theoretical knowledge linked with the testing or generating of theories through research
- *Empirical knowledge* is generated through research
- *Practical knowledge* emanates from practice; it may be generated through research or logical thought associated with practice. Many, however, would say that this type of knowledge emerges from the practice of nursing, midwifery and health visiting
- *Experiential knowledge* is accumulated through our day-to-day experiences associated with our professional and personal lives
- *Interpersonal knowledge* is linked with experiential knowledge but is associated with knowledge gained through interacting with people. This type of knowledge is particularly important within nursing, midwifery and health visiting since our practice revolves around interactions with others (patients/client, carers, peers, other professionals)
- *Ritual* is often associated with the traditions of practice and may provide a protective backdrop for care. All too often, however, the effectiveness of our rituals is unquestioned and unevaluated
- *Intuitive knowledge* is hard to define. Frequently we cannot give an explanation for it other than 'we just knew' – it appears to be the ability to come to a decision without logical thought

---

Box 3.2   A hierarchy of evidence

First item listed is ranked as highest level of evidence:

Evidence from randomised controlled trials
Evidence from controlled trials without randomisation
Evidence from cohort or case-control studies
Evidence from comparisons between times or places with/without intervention
Opinions of respected authorities (based on clinical experience), descriptive studies or reports of expert committees

Adapted from Long (1996)

- experiential
- interpersonal
- ritual
- intuitive (see Box 3.1).

Each of these also seems to have an associated value enabling a hierarchy of knowledge to be generated (Box 3.2), setting, somewhat artificially, one type (the empirical) above the rest.

The reality for many of us is that we are guided by several types of knowledge which tell us how to act in our world by informing our practice. This ensures that we are skilled and competent in order to provide appropriate care to a wide range of clients. It may, however, be the range of these types of knowledge that makes our ability to explicitly define knowledge per se so 'fuzzy', since when one asks groups of nurses, midwives or health visitors to delineate the types of knowledge that they use to inform practice, they have no difficulty in producing a list similar to the one above.

WHY DO WE NEED KNOWLEDGE?

On first consideration, the answer to this question is obvious: to provide information on which to base and build practice. However, on further exploration it is clear that practitioners use a variety of different types of knowledge, in a variety of different ways. Over the past 10 years I have asked groups of practitioners what they used knowledge for. These discussions resulted in the formation of a wide-ranging and extensive list of possibilities which go far beyond the notion of providing evidence on which to *base* practice. Rather, they suggest a use of knowledge which is associated with providing evidence to *support* practice in the widest possible sense. This allowed them, through the use of different types of knowledge, to:

- argue for resources
- present a case to other health care professionals
- inform patients/clients/carers
- improve care
- develop the discipline of nursing, midwifery or health visiting
- generate ideas for research.

In a recent research study (Mulhall et al 1996), we asked participants to describe the use of empirical knowledge in their practice; the list generated from their responses is similar to the one above and backs up the proposition that knowledge truly *supports* practice. Participants included the following as ways of using knowledge gained from research:

- to demonstrate effectiveness
- to justify skill mix
- to justify the use of bank staff
- to justify the nursing pay bill
- to improve clinical practice
- to care for the patient, or care for the environment
- to solve a problem
- to provide a rationale for practice.

This diversity suggests that practitioners use a range of knowledge from a variety of different origins, to achieve a variety of objectives.

The currency of knowledge

When we consider the different types of knowledge used in practice, there remains considerable debate surrounding the worth of each of these – their

Box 3.3 The value of evidence: impact value of various journals

Journal	Impact value	Citation index
Nature	28.417	Science
Lancet	17.948	Science
British Medical Journal	4.947	Science
Economist	12.189	Social science
Journal of Advanced Nursing	0.619	Social science
International Journal of Nursing Studies	0.330	Social science

Sources: Science Citation Index (1996), Social Science Citation Index (1996)

currency. This is evidenced by the development of hierarchies which place one mechanism for generating knowledge above another (see Box 3.2 and Chapter 6), or schemata which associate an impact value with knowledge disseminated through particular journals (Box 3.3). However, despite the availability of various hierarchical approaches and the credence given by some to these, we do not know with confidence the real value associated with each layer of any hierarchy. Foot (1974 p 84) highlights the dilemma admirably: 'One man (sic) may say that a thing is good because of some fact about it and another may refuse to take that fact as any evidence at all, for nothing is laid down in the meaning of "good" which connects it with one piece of "evidence" rather than another'.

It is clear then, that different types of knowledge have different currencies which depend on the views of those using and assessing their value. The currency of knowledge is built up in several ways which take account of the following considerations:

- the type of knowledge and its origins (Box 3.1)
- the value attributed to the type of knowledge (Box 3.2)
- the value given to different types of knowledge by different professional groupings and the power associated with these groupings
- the language used to articulate the knowledge
- the mechanism for articulating the knowledge
- others' appreciation of the knowledge being generated, exchanged and implemented
- the inherent reliability and validity of the knowledge.

Some of you will agree with the hierarchy of evidence that Long (1996) described (Box 3.2); others among you may want to tip it on its head and identify knowledge obtained from expert practitioners as central to your own practice. Perhaps, though, what we really need to do is to acknowledge the real value of knowledge *in* our practice: the actual impact of the evidence on which we base our actions. The skill, then, is not picking knowledge only from the top of a hierarchy, but rather selecting knowledge which can be applied appropriately in given situations.

The rate at which this currency can be exchanged, however, would appear to equate with the way in which the knowledge has been generated. This is aptly illustrated through the assumption that evidence can be presented hierarchically (see Box 3.2 for example) with, for some, the gold standard being that generated through experimentation. Knowledge generated in this way falls within the scientific tradition which assumes that the world in which we live is characterised by 'patterns and regularities' which we can begin to understand by logical, precise exploration, paying particular 'attention to evidence' (Schumacker & Gortner 1992 p 2). This form of knowledge – the product of traditional science – is different to knowledge generated experientially or interpersonally (see Boxes 2.1 and 8.1). Traditional scientific knowledge is believed to be 'derived from a long intellectual tradition' which has led to similarities in thinking, method and dissemination through numerous disciplines (Schumacker & Gortner 1992 p 2). Although this type of knowledge has a unique position and is valuable to the precision necessitated by skilled practice, it is not the only source of knowledge from which effective compassionate practice develops and thrives.

Knowledge derived from traditional scientific enquiries is often perceived as rather 'black or white', a quest for truth; whereas the practice of nursing, midwifery and health visiting is embedded in the more colourful elements of life, where clarity is often obscured and evidence from several sources of knowledge is required to form a solid bedrock on which to build the complexities of practice. We trust knowledge generated through the scientific tradition because we believe that it conveys a sense of truth and generalisability to evidence. This is also frequently supported by our experiences of implementing this type of knowledge and 'seeing it work'. Both of these give us a feeling of confident certainty and hope for error-free practice. But the variability of practice may still make us hesitant. We know that knowledge derived in this way, in reality, needs to be tempered by the complexities of life, health, illness or disability that our work addresses, and thus it needs to be complemented by other views of the world.

These other perspectives may be gathered through the interpretive or naturalistic traditions (see Box 8.1) which expose and value the complexities and irregularities of existence: the colourfulness of life and the impact of health, illness or disability on people and those caring for them. However, many see this type of knowledge as weak and subjective since it cannot be generalised. In hierarchies (Box 3.2), this type of data moves towards the bottom, accompanying experiential, interpersonal and intuitive knowledge.

However, increasingly there is a realisation that knowledge gained through the combination of approaches, a kaleidoscopic knowledge, may best suit the reality of practice which is typified by 'interactions between unique individuals with unique experiences...in unique situations' (Sarvimaki 1988 p 465). This provides a more realistic, all-encompassing currency to support practice. The need to combine approaches and not forsake one type of knowledge for another has been emphasised by Wilson-Barnett (1997 p 469) in her comments at a symposium on evidence-based nursing practice: 'There has been mistaken talk about a hierarchy of research which cuts out much of the work we need to do...we need to bring together the cultures of research and practice. All kinds of evidence are needed'.

It is evident then, that different sectors of the nursing, midwifery or health visiting disciplines use and value different types of knowledge and that the currency of knowledge may be affected by the social, political and economic climate of the time, since 'We cannot talk of knowing and knowledge in isolation from what we know; nor can we ignore the social significance and political consequences of that knowing' (Lawler 1997 p 34).

The combination of these factors results in an unequal allocation of a value to knowledge which depends on its origins rather than its applicability to practice. However, in reality the complexities of practice necessitate the use of different 'knowledges' or a skilled repackaging of some in order to gain acceptance by several different groups of people.

Knowledge repackaged?

Since there appears to be much controversy over the relative importance of different types of knowledge and a view that there is a gap between theory/research and practice, it is interesting to consider if knowledge is now being rebranded and sold to us in the repackaged form of evidence-based practice. We appear to be being seduced into thinking that we need something, in the form of evidence, which is different from the knowledge that we already have available to us. This repackaging is designed to revitalise our use of knowledge, in the hope that practitioners will accept the search for, and use of, evidence for their practice as a new crusade, rather than relying on ritual and tradition alone. If this is the case, then the currency of knowledge would appear to have been revalued in a move to get all health care professionals to actively consider their knowledge base in the progression towards effective, efficient and appropriate care based on the best available evidence from a variety of sources (Department of Health 1993a, 1996b).

Some naturally find the movement towards evidence-based practice confusing, believing that they were already shaping their practice in this way; others find the notion of evidence hard to grasp, aligning it to data generated through research alone rather than through a variety of different approaches (Box 3.1). However, the popularisation of the notion of evidence-based practice has captured our attention and a growth industry has developed to promote it. At present, however, this seems to stop short of acknowledging the dynamic relationship between evidence and practice, one in which evidence is refined for practice, by practice. Nursing, midwifery and health visiting are eclectic disciplines which naturally draw on different types of knowledge. This amalgam of knowledge allows us to answer the variety of questions that reflect the complexity of our work. However, in order to do this successfully, we need to articulate explicitly all types of knowledge that inform practice, rather than narrowly focusing on the inherent value of one type of knowledge over another.

If we accept the need for this refocused approach, we have to consider new ways of making our knowledge explicit, and much energy is being invested in the development of strategies to facilitate the articulation of our knowledge/evidence base in order to develop scholarship. These include:

- reflection
- analysis and discussion of critical incidents
- development of evaluative, questioning cultures
- peer review
- clinical supervision
- creation of expert panels.

Each of these, either individually or in combination, will contribute to a repackaging of our knowledge, which through appropriate dissemination will impact on practice and 'give voice to our own business' (Lawler 1997 p 49).

Alongside this considerable enterprise, the repackaging of knowledge may be occurring on a more subtle, day-to-day level, with practitioners deliberately altering the way in which they present knowledge. This alteration, or refashioning, seems to be achieved through their choice and use of language. For instance, a midwife or health visitor drawing on knowledge from a study describing women's experiences of post-natal depression may report these in a quantitative style to a natural scientist or doctor (e.g. 40% of the women in the sample felt suicidal). However, when discussing the same information with another midwife or health visitor, she or he may use a different, more qualitative style because they share a different set of values and experiences (e.g. describing the nature of the experience of feeling suicidal). It therefore appears that we need to develop skills in knowledge repackaging in order to 'sell' knowledge to others.

HOW IS KNOWLEDGE ARTICULATED AND DISSEMINATED?

Much has been written over the last decade about nurses', midwives' and health visitors' reading and publishing habits (for example Hicks 1993).

This evidence, usually accumulated through surveys, provides a picture of a profession in which members fail to disseminate information through publication, frequently under-utilise knowledge disseminated in this way and read narrowly unless they are undertaking educational courses or projects. However, this strategy fails to look at the breadth of approaches to dissemination and ways in which practitioners accumulate knowledge. In a recent phenomenological study, Mulhall et al (1996) asked 21 practitioners where they got their knowledge to practice from. Their responses showed a variety of approaches used to collect knowledge, and included the following:

- written information (journals, articles, procedure books and policies, nursing and medical notes)
- an oral tradition of passing on information from peer to peer, colleague to colleague or client to carer: 'Quite often it is hand-me-down information in the sense that it is handed down from one nurse to another' and 'Information is passed on from generation to generation and from colleague to colleague'
- formal educational opportunities
- experience
- patients
- trial and error and reflecting
- linking theory and practice through logical thought: 'Once you are able to relate theory to your practice then you are automatically able to do things'.

This diversity suggests that dissemination must be undertaken through a series of different approaches if information is to permeate the profession. Chapter 5 provides detailed information about the wide range of dissemination strategies available through print media, person-to-person contact and new technologies.

Alongside this it is interesting to note the large numbers of conferences available to nurses, midwives and health visitors, many of which remain well attended despite difficulties in securing funding and providing 'cover' to attend these events. Considering this and the comments above about passing information from generation to generation and colleague to colleague, one wonders if the most fruitful approach to dissemination and implementation of knowledge is through the oral tradition. The fact that the very essence of practice appears to revolve around interpersonal interactions and the growth of strategies to discuss practice, whereas the essence of reading and writing 'is a private activity, pursued alone and in silence...' (Warner 1994 p xi) may account for the findings of researchers who have studied the reading and writing habits of the members of our profession. One wonders if more use of the oral route for dissemination, either through formal approaches (conferences, seminars) or informally (report giving, clinical supervision, mentoring), would lead to greater critical appraisal, implementation and debate surrounding disseminated information.

Considerations related to the dissemination of knowledge

As we have already seen, not all knowledge will be disseminated formally. However, for those who do formally disseminate their knowledge, certain factors need to be considered since they will influence the process of dissemination, the likely impact of that disseminated knowledge and its effects on practice.

In 1995 the Department of Health published a document which focused on potential methods for promoting the implementation of research findings in the National Health Service (Department of Health 1995a). These ideas form a useful framework for consideration in relation to the dissemination of all knowledge, regardless of its type. In order to achieve the maximum impact, the following characteristics should be considered whenever anyone thinks that he or she has knowledge to disseminate:

- the characteristics of the message
- the characteristics of the people receiving the message
- the characteristics of the techniques being used to disseminate the message
- the levers, facilitators and barriers associated with the implementation of the message.

Under these four headings, Box 3.4 (Department of Health 1995a) gives some pointers which will help you appreciate the range of factors associated with dissemination. Some or all of these are likely to influence the success of dissemination, either formal or informal, and the likely outcome in relation to the implementation of knowledge within various practice settings.

In conjunction with these, it is important to focus on the context in which the knowledge is being exchanged and the etiquette associated with exchanging knowledge between nursing, midwifery or health visiting practitioners as well as those outside these disciplines. This exchange will vary with professional groupings, but is also likely to be affected by the individual styles of the people involved. For instance, disseminating knowledge may be achieved by openly telling someone to improve his or her practice using evidence from a particular study, or by using a more subtle approach where knowledge insidiously creeps from one practitioner to another. Griffiths & Luker (1997 p 124) provide a good example of this latter 'knowledge creep' in their discussion of the etiquette of district nursing, since for some 'It was not considered reasonable to be direct with a colleague about a patient. A more courteous approach would be to tackle the

---

Box 3.4   Factors influencing the dissemination/implementation of knowledge

Characteristics of the message

Quality
Source
Content
Presentation

Characteristics of the people receiving the message (Who are they?)

Individual health professionals (e.g. nurses, physiotherapists, speech and language therapists)
Managers (e.g. ward, unit, patch, trust, GP practice)
Purchasers of health services
Providers of health services
Partners in the provision of care (e.g. local authorities)
Professional organisations
Industry
Education providers
Research information providers
Researchers
General public
User groups
Media
Policy makers

Characteristics of the technique for dissemination

Clinical guidelines
Audit and feedback
Conferences
Local consensus processes
Educational approaches
Marketing
Opinion leaders
Reminders/computerised decision support
Patients

Levers, facilitators and barriers associated with the implementation of the message

Availability of resources
Availability of time
Financial/contractual issues
Statute
Professional incentives/disincentives
Cultural/social/organisational norms

Department of Health (1995a p 13)

---

issue indirectly...for example, some of the nurses described how they would leave journals around that contained relevant and up-to-date information about a topic; or discuss a subject in broad terms without reference to a named patient, to depersonalise the discussion'.

It may also be true to say that patients' views influence our use of knowledge. This may be achieved through shaping our knowledge to suit their individual needs or by challenging the evidence on which we base our practice. They may also criticise our use of knowledge if it leads to reduced feelings of satisfaction with the service provided, as shown by Griffiths & Luker (1997 p 125), who provide a pertinent example in this quotation from a district nurse in their study: 'They (patients) don't like it when you change things, dressings I'm thinking of, change of treatment, the way you put a bandage on. They'll tell you if somebody else goes in and does it differently'.

Griffiths & Luker (1997 p 126) found several factors that influenced district nurses' decisions to challenge colleagues about their practice, which could be considered alongside those in Box 3.4:

- whether the colleague in question was from her or his own or another team
- the personality of the colleague or relationship with the colleague
- whether the nurse believed her or his own practice to be up to date
- the patient's unknown case history
- the patient's personality
- whether challenging would damage the nurse–patient relationship
- the stress level of the substituting nurse
- the perceived seriousness of the situation
- balance between patient advocacy and respect for a colleague's autonomy.

One may deduce, therefore, that the use of knowledge does not rely on dissemination alone: it is influenced by a host of other formal and informal factors which need serious consideration.

Problems linked to dissemination

Given that we can now identify some of the factors that will make dissemination succeed or fail, it is important to spend time thinking about other problems frequently linked to dissemination. After all, knowledge can only be disseminated for implementation if some of the most commonly cited problems are acknowledged and solved. If one asks practitioners to list the most frequent reasons for the non-implementation of disseminated findings, they repeatedly focus on the following:

- unavailable or inaccessible evidence
- difficulty in understanding the language used
- inability to seek out and appraise evidence
- too much information available for synthesis and implementation
- conflicting evidence
- ambiguous findings

- the value of the information to the practice arena
- the value and impact of the information to others (such as other professional groups, clients, carers)
- the rigour of the techniques used to collect the information.

Or they simply say that the problems of implementation (e.g. resources, managing change, colleagues' attitudes) are too great to even start to overcome.

These clearly impact on a variety of different people, including those:

- generating knowledge
- disseminating knowledge
- receiving knowledge
- implementing knowledge
- supporting the dissemination of knowledge (e.g. librarians, conference organisers, educators, publishers, editors)
- supporting the implementation of knowledge (e.g. managers, practitioners, clients, carers)
- directing, through policy, the implementation of knowledge.

Knowledge, then, can only be implemented if there is support from a large group of people who have varying responsibilities throughout the dissemination–implementation continuum. The use of knowledge is therefore a complex business and this may account for some of the reluctance that surrounds the changing of practice to incorporate new knowledge.

HOW IS KNOWLEDGE IMPLEMENTED?

It is probably fair to say that we implement knowledge that is relevant to our practice every minute of the working day. This knowledge has been generated through a variety of different routes (Box 3.1), disseminated, appraised and implemented; dissemination alone does not mean that knowledge will be implemented. Yet much of this process of implementation goes unnoticed with few of us thinking too much about it. In the main, implementation of knowledge is generally invisible and as such forms part of skilled, effective practice. However, this changes when we implement new knowledge: in these instances the process becomes more visible since it necessitates the management of change and the complexities that accompany it. Both Chapters 8 and 9 provide valuable information and insight into this process.

What will encourage the implementation of disseminated knowledge?

Entwistle et al (1996) suggest a variety of approaches which may lead to the implementation of disseminated knowledge, including:

Box 3.5   Key features of disseminated knowledge

- Relevance: the information must be relevant to the decision being made
- Comprehensiveness: is all the necessary information provided?
- Accuracy: does the information reflect the best available evidence?
- Accessibility: can the information be obtained easily?
- Comprehensibility: is the information understandable?
- Acceptability: is the proposed care acceptable to clients/patients/carers?

Entwistle et al (1996)

- disseminating information in a variety of ways
- supporting continuing professional development
- designing clinical guidelines
- sending reminders
- issuing policy statements
- specifying practice requirements in contracts
- facilitating financial incentives.

Any or all of these will also need to be combined with the certainty that the knowledge is relevant, comprehensive, accurate, understandable, acceptable and accessible (Entwistle et al 1996) (Box 3.5) if implementation is to occur. To do this, practitioners need to develop sophisticated skills associated with the retrieval, appraisal and synthesis of knowledge to enable them to determine the 'worth' of the knowledge presented to them. This is particularly important since the amount of knowledge available has mushroomed over the last 30 years, and is likely to continue to do so. In these circumstances one cannot simply presume that all disseminated knowledge is sound and relevant and will be effective or efficient if utilised. A decision needs to be made about the 'worth' of the knowledge coupled with an assessment of its 'clinical relevance' and transferability from the setting in which the original knowledge was generated to that in which the practitioner plans to use the knowledge.

One constant problem, since our knowledge requires continual fine tuning through updating, is the amount of disseminated information that practitioners can store and keep up with. This dilemma has recently resulted in an emphasis on the use of systematic reviews of evidence. These are designed to provide clear, unbiased summaries of evidence which answer clinically relevant questions (see Chapter 6). Although this approach may encourage the use of disseminated knowledge simply because it is made into an easily manageable form, care must be taken to appraise the review and determine the clinical relevance of the outcome(s) suggested for practice. Careful evaluation of the usefulness of this approach needs to take place. How much knowledge is implemented as a result of this technique, and what is its impact on the retrieval and appraisal abilities of practitioners? One hopes that a technique designed to increase effectiveness and efficiency will not deskill nurses, midwives and health visitors in using techniques (of retrieving, appraising and synthesising knowledge) that many are only now becoming competent and confident in using.

Even with all of these problems solved, the real and complex demands of practice may stand in the way of implementation, and further opportunities may need to be provided. Le May et al (1997) found that practitioners felt that they needed a battery of supportive opportunities to implement knowledge generated through research. These included:

- increased levels of support from colleagues and managers
- reduced resistance from colleagues from their own and other's disciplines
- consolidation of new knowledge
- the existence of role models to follow.

as well as their own need to become:

- more persistent
- more educated
- more independent.

Knowledge, through implementation, is at risk of losing its purity as it is sullied by the realities of practice and is thus changing its complexion. Implementation may alter knowledge in a bizarre way, since in some instances the knowledge revered for practice becomes, through the process of implementation, a burden, due to the complexity of the change process required to move it into the practice arena. The implementation of knowledge is a skilled venture requiring forethought and careful change management (see Chapter 8).

CONCLUSION

The types of knowledge used influence the language of dissemination and the extent to which knowledge impacts on practice. There is little use in continuing to generate new knowledge unless it leads to changes in practice that benefit the providers and users of nursing, midwifery and health visiting services, thus leading to clinical effectiveness. Knowledge in a vacuum is fruitless, whereas knowledge used to enhance practice is of the utmost importance.

Nursing knowledge is no longer a certainty handed down from generation to generation; it is dynamic, uncertain and growing. In order to keep pace with this, we rely on skilled dissemination drawing on the variety of types of knowledge to provide an accurate, accessible bedrock for use by an eclectic discipline.

4

Perceptions of research

Anne Lacey

KEY POINTS

- Nurses and professions allied to medicine are relative newcomers to a research culture
- Quantitative studies measuring attitudes towards research show nurses to have a positive attitude, but this does not necessarily translate into behaviour that promotes research-based practice
- Qualitative studies provide some clues as to why research implementation is often slow
- Apart from the medical profession, attitudes towards research and its implementation are very similar across all groups of health professionals
- Health practitioners lack confidence in their research skills, and are reluctant to publish and disseminate their work
- Managerial attitudes are sometimes unsupportive towards those health professionals who do wish to pursue a research agenda
- Nurses need to become more willing to share with and learn from other professions, particularly those using social science research

---

INTRODUCTION

Research and development are high on the agenda of the National Health Service (NHS), particularly since the Culyer Report (Department of Health 1994a) and its subsequent adoption within the NHS Research and Development (R & D) strategy. Output from the Department of Health, as well as the professional bodies, emphasises the need for 'evidence-based practice' and for practitioners to be research-aware (Department of Health 1991, 1993b, 1994c). There is an assumption in much of such literature that bodies of research-based knowledge exist which are relevant to health care practitioners, and that this research is continually being added to and refined. The emphasis is on how to get such knowledge into practice.

How do practitioners themselves view research, however? Is it a reality in the clinical environment, or an irrelevance that rarely impinges on the everyday round of patient care? These questions will be the basis of this chapter.

HOW DO PRACTITIONERS VIEW RESEARCH?

Perceptions among nurses

Several recent studies have been carried out among British nurses, and most have found that overall, attitudes to research are generally positive, but this does not necessarily lead on to the ready use of research findings. Pearcey (1995) surveyed 600 nurses and nurse tutors by questionnaire, achieving a 67% response rate. Of the sample, 78% agreed that research findings could improve care (or teaching), agreement being strongest among those most recently trained. Those who had been trained over 20 years were least likely to agree that research was useful. Night staff were also less likely to have a positive attitude towards research. There was much evidence of dissatisfaction with respondents' own research skills, less than 10% considering that these were adequate. Perceived needs were wide-ranging, including locating research, reading it critically, applying it to practice, and sharing knowledge. Pearcey concludes that nurses lack confidence in research because of the lack of emphasis on it in pre-registration training.

Veeramah (1995) carried out a questionnaire survey among 150 mental health practitioners in the south of England. A 78% response rate was achieved. This was one of a small number of studies focused on the mental health area, but showed results remarkably similar to those carried out in other clinical settings. A very positive attitude towards research was found, but the majority of nurses felt that they did not have the necessary skills to interpret research findings critically or to apply them to practice. Furthermore, 81% felt that they needed some or a lot of help in making use of research findings.

It is disappointing to find that, despite the nurses' positive attitude as shown in the sample, a large proportion do not use research findings to a large extent in practice. What can be deduced from the rest of the findings is that a positive attitude towards research is a significant and necessary variable but is not in itself sufficient to influence the use of research findings in practice. (Veeramah 1995 p 859)

However, I believe that there has at least been a change in attitude since the early 1980s when writers such as Hunt (1981) considered that nurses were negative in their attitude towards research.

Nelson (1995), working in Scotland, discusses the need to develop a research culture among nurses in the UK. He considers the necessity for each practitioner to become research-aware in order to fulfil the requirements of the professional body for accountability. He investigated the extent to which action research projects undertaken by post-basic students were being utilised, and found some resistance to change by those not personally involved in the projects. In particular, nurse managers who were unsupportive could be obstructive in the translation of research into practice.

The development of a research culture, in particular support by clinical managers, is a major factor in research utilisation ... lack of peer support, in conjunction with the expectation that research is never or only an occasionally expected activity in their unit, indicates the absence of a research culture within clinical areas. (Nelson 1995 p 188)

This issue will be discussed in more detail later. Nelson also discovered a lack of confidence among respondents regarding their research skills, and discusses the need for 'user-friendly' research.

Experience in the UK is not dissimilar to that in the rest of the world. Research from Israel by Eckerling et al (1988) suggests a link between educational level and research attitudes and ability. This study measured attitudes and abilities in research among university nursing students, from undergraduate to doctoral level. Perceptions of ability in research were found to be closely linked to attitude, those having most confidence in their research abilities showing the most positive attitudes towards it. Attitude and ability had a major impact on each other, and influenced perceptions of the nurse's role. Those with greater confidence in their own research abilities also tended to see research as integral to their role, and were often among the most highly educated section of the sample. So confidence is very closely bound up with attitudes towards research, as is echoed in many writings on the subject.

In Australia, Wright et al (1996) surveyed 410 general and psychiatric nurses in hospital and community practice using a questionnaire. Again, a positive attitude towards research was found, but this did not correlate with use of research in practice. Whereas 91% believed nursing research to be necessary, only 73% saw a need for it in their own clinical area. 'RN's believe research should occur "out there" – but not where it will involve them' (Wright et al 1996 p 18). Again, many respondents identified a need for education in research, expressing dissatisfaction with the extent to which research education was covered in their basic training. No significant differences were found in the value attributed to research between nurses from different educational backgrounds or different clinical settings.

In summary, research suggests that:

- Nurses are generally positive in their attitude towards research
- Nurses find research difficult to read and evaluate
- Nurses trained more recently find it easier to access and use research
- Nurses are dissatisfied about their own research skills
- Managers do not always facilitate a 'research culture'.

Perceptions among specialisms within the nursing professions

Nurses' attitudes towards research cannot be viewed in isolation from the other professions with whom they work. Even within nursing, health visiting and midwifery there are differences as regards the status and traditions of research. Early research was concentrated on hospital-based acute specialities, although there were notable exceptions such as Hockey's well-described and honest account of research in the community (Hockey 1985). Mental health and learning disability branches of nursing find themselves with a smaller body of research with which to work, and little by way of definitive findings that can be implemented directly. By the nature of work in these areas, research tends to be exploratory and qualitative, although in the field of behavioural therapies some experimental research is available, often conducted by social scientists and psychologists rather than nurses themselves. Earlier in the chapter we noted the work of Veeramah (1995) which illustrated that nurses in the area of mental health, while holding positive attitudes were, like general nurses, less concerned with implementing research.

A commendably large body of midwife-led research has been developed during recent years, but research indicates that in common with nursing, the weight of tradition militates against the adoption of evidence-based practice (Harris 1992). Midwifery has been able to develop a range of research styles, from qualitative work exploring the experience of childbirth (Bluff & Holloway 1994, Walker et al 1995) to case-controlled trials about neural tube defects (Wright 1995).

With regard to research utilisation in midwifery, similar results have been obtained to those for nurses. Hicks (1993) conducted a questionnaire survey using a national random sample of 550 midwives in England, Scotland and Wales, obtaining a 72% response rate. She found attitudes towards research broadly positive, midwives seeing research as having an important role to play within their profession. The most commonly cited obstacles to research included lack of time, knowledge and confidence, but midwives did not see research as irrelevant to their role. She describes midwives as 'diffident' in their attitude to research; they valued it, but felt under-confident in engaging in research skills. This diffidence leads to a limited number of publications being produced by midwives, and hence to a small research base in the literature. Hicks found that possession of a post-basic qualification was the most important determinant of involvement in research activity, these midwives being more likely to initiate research, gain funding and submit their work for publication. Presumably the confidence gained from a post-basic course goes some way to persuading midwives that they are capable of producing reputable research.

Earlier work by Hicks (1992) also suggests that midwives may lack confidence in their own credibility as researchers. In an experimental study, midwives rated research less favourably when they believed it was carried out by a midwife researcher than when they believed it to have been done by an obstetrician. Again, confidence emerges as the key factor that is lacking, inhibiting the health professions from emerging into a truly research-based profession. 'What appears to emerge from this is fairly unequivocal evidence that the principle issue which prevents midwives from initiating research and presumably its subsequent dissemination is one of a crisis of confidence, about their ability either to undertake good quality research or to submit it for publication' (Hicks 1993 p 60).

ATTITUDES TOWARDS RESEARCH IN OTHER HEALTH PROFESSIONS

The medical profession

The dominant profession of medicine has, of course, long held a monopoly in research in the Health Service. Being built, as it is, on a scientific discipline that has depended for much of its knowledge on laboratory and clinical empirical work, medical research has been held in high esteem by the public since the beginning of the NHS, and has been funded accordingly. 'Teaching' hospitals were those that had a medical school, and hence a university base and research-active staff. Such hospitals had high prestige as centres of excellence and many had additional funding from charitable institutions and trust funds. The majority of government funds for health research were channelled through these institutions and were managed by the medical profession. The Culyer Report (Department of Health 1994a) has at last provided a fairer system whereby research funding can be accessed by other professions and by non-teaching hospitals, as well as by practitioners in community and primary care. Possession is, however, nine-tenths of the law. Those institutions that already have well-established research centres and the staff and other resources required are likely to still get the lion's share of the funds available. The public, in addition, view 'medical research' very favourably and readily contribute to charities researching sensitive conditions such as cancer and meningitis. Medical research is dominated by the 'gold standard' of the randomised controlled trial. This method of research is valued as being objective, scientific and the best way of measuring clinical effectiveness. The current drive for 'evidence-based' health care subscribes to this view, and medical research is therefore advantaged in status. There is much medical research that does not follow this pattern, however, including some epidemiological designs, case studies and the growing fields of outcomes research and audit. Quantitative methods still predominate in medicine, and until very recently qualitative methods were dismissed as unscientific and lacking in rigour (Pope & Mays 1995).

Attitudes towards research among medical practitioners are more difficult to describe as there is little, if any, research into this area. The actual conduct of major research is restricted to a small elite within the profession, but many others are involved in recruiting to, and collecting data for, multi-centre trials that are managed by remote research centres, often on an international level. Medical education has been university-based for many decades, and its practitioners are expected to practice autonomously, taking responsibility for their own professional development. It is not frowned upon for medical practitioners to take time during their working hours to read professional journals, see representatives of pharmaceutical companies, or to attend lectures that are available in their workplace. The organisation of a hospital doctor's working day allows her or him to fit in time for study if the 'bleep' allows. Recent reports about discrepancies in treatment, however, suggest that not all doctors keep themselves abreast of the most recent research findings (e.g. Little et al 1996). Even where they are aware of new practices, they may choose to ignore research findings that suggest that traditional methods of surgery, for example, are disadvantageous. Nurses in several studies, including my own (Lacey 1994) have cited doctors as a barrier to research implementation, for example, surgeons may insist on traditional methods of preparation for theatre even when research suggests that these are inappropriate. Several papers have been published recently that suggest that increasing proportions of medical interventions are evidence-based (Ellis et al 1995, Gill et al 1996), but the definition of 'evidence-based' remains contentious (Greenhalgh 1996).

Certain fields of medicine have not developed such a strong research base, and these include primary care. Here medical practitioners are working in teams with other health professionals and could gain much from collaborative research, but the randomised controlled trial may not be the ideal research method (Greenhalgh 1996). Funding for primary care research has not been readily available until the recent changes following the Culyer Report (Department of Health 1994a).

In summary, the research tradition in medicine is characterised thus:

- medicine has its root in scientific disciplines that use laboratory research
- medical schools are located in universities
- medical research has a high public profile and is well funded
- medical practitioners are able to combine research with clinical practice
- medicine is the dominant health profession, and sets much of the agenda in NHS research.

The professions allied to medicine

The professions allied to medicine (physiotherapy, occupational therapy, radiography, podiatry, speech and language therapy) are in a very different position from medicine as regards research, having in many instances more in common with nursing and midwifery. Recent government reports (Department of Health 1993b, 1994c) have discussed ways in which these professions may best be enabled to contribute to the NHS R & D strategy.

There is little empirical evidence of the extent of utilisation of research in these professions, or of attitudes towards research among practitioners. One study (Challen et al 1996) does address these issues for the radiography profession, but for the following discussion I have also drawn on opinion articles and several years of contact with both colleagues and students in the therapy professions.

The therapy professions have, within the last decade, moved from training resulting in a professional diploma to graduate status. Although many have been located within higher education for some years (but usually within the old polytechnic sector rather than the traditional universities), the training was governed by the professional bodies who emphasised practical competency; until recently there was little training in research. This has necessarily changed with the introduction of graduate entry, and there is now a growing pool of newly qualified members of each of the therapy professions who have some experience of doing research for their own qualifications, and who have been trained to access research and question clinical practice.

This is not without its problems; for example, experienced podiatrists using treatment methods taught during their own training do not necessarily welcome inexperienced newcomers who introduce a research study which brings established practice into question. This is a common problem across all the professions, including nursing: where educational preparation for practice is changed, those in relatively senior positions without the new qualifications are bound to feel defensive and may resent well-qualified but inexperienced practitioners who attempt to put forward new and challenging ideas. Nurses trained under Project 2000 express similar difficulties (see Chapter 7). Many ward sisters are anxious that the newly trained nurses may have plenty of 'head knowledge' but inadequate practical experience to render them safe practitioners. Some traditionally trained practitioners hold the belief that academic study somehow makes people unfit for practical competence, that the two cannot work together to produce a 'knowledgeable doer', as the Project 2000 document put it (United Kingdom Central Council for Nursing, Midwifery and Health Visiting 1986). None of this is new; as a student on one of the first nursing degree courses in the 1970s, I and my colleagues encountered a lot of prejudice and at times downright hostility from both senior staff and fellow students on the traditional training courses. There was a fear that graduate nurses would expect to take over senior positions immediately after qualifying, and that the very fact that we had studied for a degree meant we were unlikely to make 'good nurses'. Until this anti-academic culture within the professions is dispelled, we are unlikely to make much progress towards the research-based professions to which all claim to aspire.

Challen et al's (1996) study of radiographers found, in common with many studies in nursing, a positive attitude towards research in principle.

This study used a quantitative approach, sending a questionnaire to a convenience sample of 185 radiographers in a single geographical area of the UK. The response rate achieved was only 55%, so the results must be viewed with some caution; it could be that those with more negative attitudes towards research also had negative attitudes towards filling in postal questionnaires! Almost two-thirds of respondents had been involved in some research activity, some more newly qualified as part of their degree programme, but others as part of a wider research team. Respondents generally viewed research as a good thing, but only 21% thought of it as a professional requirement. Deterrents to research were similar to those in other professions: lack of knowledge and time were the principle problems. There was a reluctance to publish research: none of the respondents had published the work in which they had been involved.

Lack of confidence appears to be a besetting problem for all the non-medical professions as regards dissemination of the admittedly small amount of research that is being conducted. Most of the professions allied to medicine have only one or two journals specific to their own profession, and must 'borrow' material from other disciplines. Indeed the status of the smaller professions like podiatry is such that academics seeking to bolster their publication records frequently publish in medical journals rather than those specific to their own profession. Consequently, practitioners may never see the research relevant to their own profession.

Robinson (1993) likens nurses and other caring professionals to the geographers and pharmacists in Becher's (1989) study of the nature of academic disciplines. Such disciplines are characterised by multidisciplinarity and heterogeneity within the profession, resulting in a dilution of academic knowledge specific to the discipline and a lack of academic prestige. A weak theory base specific to the discipline results in a tendency to adopt uncritically the methods and language from other, more established, disciplines. This sounds very familiar when we consider the concern of many of the professions allied to medicine to gain credibility by using 'hard' scientific research methods such as the randomised controlled trial borrowed from medical science. The professions allied to medicine are generally in a weaker position than nursing and midwifery in relation to developing their own body of research-based knowledge. Sheer lack of numbers, and the relative newness of research as part of the professional agenda, means that the amount of literature specific to each profession is small. In many cases, research can be utilised from other professions without difficulty.

Medicine and nursing both have a large overlap in their concerns with the therapy professions, in areas such as tissue viability, pain and rehabilitation, for example. In such areas, research carried out by one professional group can be directly used by another, although the emphasis may be slightly different. In other areas, research is less generalisable. I recently supervised a podiatry student who was researching the relative efficacy of different local anaesthetic agents in foot surgery, but the only comparable literature came from dentistry. The soft tissues of the oral cavity are somewhat different from the bony structures within the foot in their response to local anaesthetics! So there is a concern to build up specific literature within each of the therapy professions, but this will take time. The reluctance to publish documented by Challen et al (1996) must be overcome if this is to be achieved, and the underlying lack of confidence in research skills addressed. Craik (1997), writing about occupational therapy, mentions the lack of appropriately qualified supervisors for postgraduate studies in the specific professional field of the smaller professions, and echoes Challen et al's concern about the reluctance of practitioners to publish their work.

Nursing, in contrast, has a wealth of journals available to it, but many are seen as inaccessible to the clinical practitioner, and those of a 'lighter' style may not carry very much by way of actual research. There is little incentive to spend precious off-duty time writing up an article for publication if this is not valued when it comes to job promotion prospects. Only those employed in academic institutions therefore have the necessity to publish to maintain their credibility, and this perpetuates the perception in the professions that research is something beyond the scope of clinical practice, and is best left to academics and professional researchers.

Research in the therapy professions seems at the moment to be predominantly quantitative in nature. This is perhaps less so for the more social science-based professions such as occupational therapy, but is certainly true for radiography and podiatry and, to a lesser extent, physiotherapy. These professions have a strong base in the natural sciences of biology, physics and physiology, and naturally turn to traditional research methods used in science such as laboratory experiments. Since medicine already has a strong research base in the quantitative field, the therapy professions may find it easier to gain approval for research and funding if they are using methods acceptable to the dominant profession. Similarly, many practitioners will have been involved, perhaps as data collectors, in medical research studies which used quantitative methods. If the profession is struggling to gain recognition for its research base, qualitative methods may be seen as an unnecessary risk.

Perhaps one solution to this difficulty would be for the therapy professions, in common with the nursing professions, to recognise their natural base in the social as well as the biomedical sciences. All health professionals are dealing with people in the same way as are social workers, counsellors, educationalists and other caring professions. These professions are similarly struggling for professional status and a wider research base, but have tended to use a broader range of methods drawn from disciplines in the social and behavioural sciences. Here there is a strong tradition of research using eclectic methods from which the health professions could learn and with which they could identify. We will return to this theme in the conclusion to this chapter.

In summary, research in the professions allied to medicine is characterised by:

- the recent move to graduate status
- its low impact until the last decade
- the small body of knowledge and lack of academic prestige specific to each discipline
- a lack of confidence to publish among practitioners
- the specialist nature of journals
- older practitioners and managers who are often resistant to change.

MEASURING ATTITUDES TOWARDS RESEARCH

Most research into attitudes has been quantitative in nature, typically using questionnaires with Likert-type scales. Champion & Leach (1989) developed a questionnaire which has been modified and used by others, including those in the UK (Lacey 1994, Veeramah 1995). They attempted to identify variables related to research utilisation, including attitude, availability and support. Attitude to research was tested by a series of statements such as 'Understanding research helps me practise nursing professionally', 'Research is a dull boring subject', with which respondents are invited to indicate their strength of agreement or disagreement on a five-point scale. The study, originally carried out in a single hospital in America, showed attitude and availability of research findings to be the most significant factors in determining research utilisation. Most of the studies carried out recently in the UK have measured research attitudes in a similar way, including a small pilot study which I conducted myself (Lacey 1994). It is possible, however, that the validity of such a measuring tool may be compromised. We know that research is associated with feelings of anxiety and guilt by many nurses (Perkins 1992). It is likely, then, that when confronted with a questionnaire about attitudes towards, and use of, research in practice, nurses may be less than honest in their responses. Social desirability may encourage responses that show a positive attitude because, as we have seen, a research base is an implicit requirement of professional practice. To admit that practice is *not* based on research may be tantamount to confessing professional malpractice. This is not to suggest that nurses are likely to lie deliberately in response to surveys, but self-report is not always the most reliable guide to behaviour or attitudes.

Other research studies, then, have used more qualitative methods to explore attitudes towards research. Rodgers (1994) conducted an exploratory study of research utilisation among nurses in Scotland, prior to a larger, quantitative study. She gathered data by means of informal discussions and interviews with staff from general medical and surgical wards. By this means, Rodgers hoped to gain insight into clinical nurses' perceptions of factors affecting research utilisation. Attitudes were not 'measured' in this qualitative study, but are revealed by some of the data reported. Nurses expressed views that research findings were not highly regarded, especially if they were at variance with their normal practice. In explaining lack of research utilisation, respondents commented on the tendency to continue with existing practices despite research evidence that might be to the contrary. Lip service was paid to the importance of research, but practical caring was somehow separated from this. Rodgers quotes from one of her interviews: 'People will say they believe in something, or they would like a certain type of care for themselves or one of their family but then do something very different (for a patient). There seems to be two sides of the brain, one thinks, one does' (Rodgers 1994 p 909). She also identified a great fear of making mistakes, and therefore a reluctance to innovate. It is 'safer' to follow routine than to question and open oneself up to criticism by adopting new practices based on one's own reading of research.

Meah et al (1996) explored midwives' attitudes towards research using small focus groups of midwives from several NHS trusts in north-west England to produce qualitative data. In common with Hicks (1993), they found a consensus among their respondents that research was highly relevant to midwifery practice, but again difficulties were expressed in accessing and interpreting research findings. There was a perception that younger, more recently trained midwives had the skills to access research, whereas those who had been trained some years ago were lacking in the skills of literature searching and critical reading. One respondent admitted that there was probably a third group who, as experienced midwives, had picked up the research skills for themselves. Statistics presented particular difficulties and real fears for many respondents.

Perkins (1992) discusses her perceptions, based on many years of teaching research skills, that nurses are afraid of research. There is an idea that research is done by 'clever' people and written in language that is difficult to understand. It is perceived as necessarily bound up with statistical techniques that instil fear in most nurses. There is also a belief that understanding research implies a necessity to criticise the work of others, which is not seen as congruent with the culture within nursing. Although not a research study, Perkins' work attempts to use qualitative discussion to get behind the reasons why nurses, although professing to be positive towards research, have such difficulty in using it. Table 4.1 illustrates the major differences between qualitative and quantitative approaches to research.

In my own study, I decided to add a qualitative semi-structured interview to my quantitative measure of research utilisation and attitudes. In this way it was hoped to 'scratch beneath the surface' of socially and professionally constructed responses, and elicit more deep-seated responses.

Table 4.1 Major differences between quantitative and qualitative research

Quantitative	Qualitative
Data are numerical	Data are in words/observations
Uses questionnaires/measurements	Uses interviews/unstructured methods
Statistical analysis	Thematic/content analysis
Large scale, generalisable	Smaller scale, in-depth
Tests relationships, explains	Explores, describes phenomena

Firstly, it seemed important to ensure that nurses (in this case, F and G grade nurses working in general adult hospital wards) understood the meaning of the word 'research'. I asked respondents if they could define research: very few could, on being asked such a question with no advance warning. Several were able to summon appropriate words such as 'hypothesis', 'critical investigation', 'systematic', demonstrating a knowledge of research terminology, and others were able to discuss different approaches to research such as randomised controlled trials or qualitative research. Some, however, included theoretical concepts such as nursing models within the definition of research, seeing almost anything that was printed in a journal as constituting research. This calls into question the validity of quantitative surveys which use the word 'research' to measure attitudes. A nurse's attitude towards nursing models may be very different from her or his attitude towards empirical research. When it came to giving examples of where research was used in practice, however, all the nurses were able to cite practice that was based on research, although they rarely knew the exact study in question.

Both the qualitative and quantitative data indicated that attitudes towards research were favourable, but the realities of implementation meant that research often acquired negative associations. Many nurses, for example, expressed frustration that they were unable to access research for themselves. This was due to both lack of time and physical access to a library, as well as an inability to understand and evaluate research once it was available. Going to the library, even if a satisfactory one was available on site, was not perceived as something that could be done legitimately in 'work time'. Consequently, any desire to look up research on a clinical issue had to be pursued during off-duty time or study days, where these were available. Unless a nurse had trained at the hospital in which she or he was working, she or he was often unfamiliar with the information systems available in the library and lacked the confidence to find out more. Information technology in the form of CD-ROM databases have an aura of mystery to the uninitiated, and even computerised library catalogues can be enough to deter use of the library.

Moreover, nurses felt they lacked the critical reading skills necessary to use research reports even if they managed to access them. Not only are there likely to be complicated tables of statistics and use of unfamiliar jargon, but the confidence to implement recommendations of a report in one's own area of practice is often lacking. Without considerable research skills training, it is difficult to know if a piece of work is valid, and whether it will generalise to other geographical or clinical areas. Implementation may require negotiation with managers or other professional groups such as doctors, and considerable confidence is required in such a context if change is to be brought about. Lack of autonomy was seen as a barrier to research utilisation, again suggesting some negative perceptions about research even though basic attitudes were positive. Overall there was a feeling of 'we would if we could' – a sense of powerlessness was associated with the knowledge that practice should be research based (see Chapter 8 for a further discussion of power).

Two factors were commonly cited as helping to reduce this sense of frustration. The first was the provision of specialist resource persons who were usually, but not necessarily, nurses. These were facilitators who could make research accessible by reading and predigesting it, translating it into workable recommendations for practice which were research based. So a tissue viability nurse might provide a guide to appropriate dressings for different kinds of wound, citing the relevant research studies but obviating the need for every nurse to read them. Such a human resource could also be relied upon to evaluate the research studies and keep clinical staff up to date. The second factor that helped in producing a more positive feeling about research was the provision of educational courses and study days. Although not necessarily about research, these courses provided enough relief from day-to-day pressures and time to reflect to encourage participants to access and use research. In addition, course members were often required to engage in a literature review or carry out a small piece of research which resulted in implications for change in practice. This may involve more than the participants themselves as they return to the ward to share their new ideas. Several informants in my research said something to the effect of: 'Well it started when Jane went on a course'.

So qualitative approaches to the study of attitudes towards research reveal a more complex picture than that elicited through quantitative studies. Nurses may well, as the majority of quantitative studies reveal, be favourable towards research in general, but when it comes to translating that favourable attitude into practice, difficulties are encountered that tend to prevent them from wholeheartedly embracing a research culture. 'Learned helplessness' (Seligman 1975) may mean that an enthusiastic foray to the library that ended in frustration and failure will result in a reluctance and even fear of trying such a venture again. Dismissive words from a senior nurse or other professional may dash confidence to share research findings with others. An encounter with an over-confident student nurse who quotes names and dates of research articles to suggest that existing practices are antiquated, if not downright dangerous, may put an anxious ward sister on the defensive.

HOW DO WE MAKE RESEARCH A CLINICAL REALITY?
Education and training

The discussion thus far indicates that progress in changing attitudes, and especially in developing confidence in research in the nursing and other professions, is vital. Education and training are obvious ways of achieving this, particularly for practitioners who have not developed research skills in their initial training for registration. The *Report of the Task Force on the Strategy for Research in Nursing Midwifery and Health Visiting* (Department of Health 1993b) acknowledges that research skills and experience need to be far more widespread than at present in the nursing profession, and that continuing education is needed to address this need. ' "Catch-up" courses are required to enable established practitioners and managers to deepen their understanding of research processes and the utilisation of research findings. More opportunities are also required for them to become acquainted with the latest research findings and to contribute to linking research and practice at every stage from that of research problem definition to that of research based service development' (Department of Health 1993b p 13).

One such course that I have been involved with as a university lecturer for some years is the English National Board for Nursing, Midwifery and Health Visiting (ENB) 870, Introduction to the Understanding and Application of Research. In 1994, an evaluation to assess lasting changes in attitudes and practice was undertaken for one cohort 6 months after completion of the course. This evaluation has been disseminated more fully elsewhere (Lacey 1996), but a few points are of relevance here. One of the skills most frequently identified in the literature (e.g. Armitage 1990, Harris 1992) as enabling research utilisation is the confident reading and critiquing of research. Six months after the course, written evaluations showed how this skill had changed perceptions of the utility of research to clinical practice. Typical comments included:

I am more careful and read a piece of research critically before advocating a change in practice.
I am more likely to look for research on areas in practice.
I am more confident in finding my own research to back up theories/practices I want to introduce.

Learning research and critical reading skills gave practitioners the crucial confidence to use research knowledge as part and parcel of their practice, it no longer being seen as something alien or for academics only.

Similarly, an educational course can give practitioners the confidence to believe that change in practice can be achieved, and this acts as a spur to initiate change. The ENB 870 course that I have been involved with requires students to develop a proposal for research-based change that can be implemented in their own area of practice. Six months after completion of the course, we asked students whether they had been able to implement their proposals. Of those who responded, 65% had been able to implement the proposal to some extent. Others had also used the proposal but fell short of implementation, or still hoped to achieve implementation in the future. Those who had been unable to use their proposals cited two sets of constraining factors: lack of seniority and therefore autonomy to make the changes; and management/organisational changes that were preventing constructive developments at the present time.

A recent study carried out in the Trent region (Brooker et al 1996) throws some light on the constraints that hinder the development of research skills in practice. In 1994 the Department of Health, concerned about the availability of appropriately trained researchers in different professions to take forward the R & D strategy, funded a study to examine the difficulties experienced by clinicians and managers who sought to develop their research skills (Department of Health 1994a). This research was conducted by the Sheffield Centre for Health and Related Research, and covered all the health professions including medicine. A questionnaire was sent to all applicants for research training in Trent during 1993–1994 (n = 292), and a 66% response rate was obtained. Research training could be full- or part-time, often involving registering for an academic qualification such as a higher degree. The sample included doctors, dentists, nurses, members of several therapy professions, and full-time researchers. The composition of the sample was interesting in itself, as these were self-selected applicants who felt in need of developing their research skills. There was a very strong community focus, with 12% from general practice/community backgrounds, 11% from maternal/child health, 9.4% from mental health and 7.3% from public health. Together these groups made up 40% of the sample, and the vast majority of those still engaged in clinical work. Nearly 75% of the sample was female, the largest professional group being nurses.

Respondents consistently rated the frustrating process of applying for funding as the most important difficulty in pursuing research training in the NHS, including the uncertainties about why some proposals were accepted and others turned down. The next difficulty was loss of income and clinical expertise while engaged in full-time research/training. In these items all the professional groups concurred. Significant differences between groups were found, however, when it came to managerial support for research training. Nurses and the therapy professions encountered significantly less supportive attitudes from managers in requesting research training than did doctors, dentists and full-time researchers. If they were given time to engage in research training, managers were more resistant if extra resources were required to engage a locum to cover the respondent's absence. Consequently there were comments such as 'I have to fit 5 days work into 4 days'. Furthermore, unless the respondents were physically separated from the clinical environment, they found that clinical priorities always took precedence and research time was 'squeezed out'.

The report concludes that one of the main obstacles to gaining such training in the NHS is the attitude of managers, who need a greater appreciation of the potential of research. A change in the culture of trusts is required, as employers tend to see full-time academic study as deskilling. One respondent said: 'Employers see full-time academic study as a loss of ability, not an increase in knowledge and skills'. Furthermore, in the nursing and therapy professions, peers are an obstacle to the development of research skills, as they do not see research as 'real work' and so are unsupportive of colleagues requiring time away from clinical responsibilities (Chapter 8 includes a further discussion of these issues).

Managers and the development of a research culture

The Trent region research discussed above underlines the importance of attitudes towards research in determining the extent to which a 'research culture' can be fostered. Key personnel such as managers can effectively block the development of practitioners who see research as important, but lack the confidence in their own research skills to engage in research or implement research findings in their own clinical sphere. The Report of the Task Force on the Strategy for Research concurs with this finding: 'Research and the change processes involved in deploying research findings must themselves be supported by a managerial culture which genuinely values research as a means of pursuing the corporate goal of health gain. This is true for the whole of the NHS R & D strategy. Our evidence suggests that neither the managerial culture in the National Health Service nor the nursing practice culture has been sufficiently supportive' (Department of Health 1993b p 11).

If managers are to be convinced of the value of research in today's cost-conscious NHS, however, they must see it as delivering results in terms of improved patient care. Academic research that gains credit for the researcher but then 'sits on the shelf' is of no use in meeting targets for efficiency or quality assurance. So research has to be implemented and translated into clinical practice that produces measurable results. English (1994) underlines this point:

'For nursing research to play any role in the future of health care, researchers must convince health care managers that nursing research deserves investment not only for the aspirations of the nursing profession but also for the continued quality of patient care. Senior decision makers may not be sympathetic to nursing issues and may be looking for returns for the investment. Unless research has a pragmatic value in the workplace, it will be perceived as being irrelevant to managers. If it is irrelevant, it is expendable' (English 1994 p 405).

CONCLUSION

Researchers in all the health professions, then, need to overcome their reluctance, their fear of criticism and their lack of confidence alongside their medical colleagues, and press ahead with relevant clinical research. Having carried out the research, the findings need to be published and disseminated through a number of channels so that the professions as a whole can access the knowledge and implement the findings (see Chapter 5 for a discussion of dissemination strategies). To foster this, however, at least some practitioners need to be given the appropriate education and research skills training, and subsequently the facility within their clinical work to develop a research active role. Managers and fellow professionals will need to enlarge their vision sufficiently to see the value of this work and its potential as a long-term investment in improving patient care and the status of the health professions.

Furthermore, the health professions need to become more eclectic in their traditions. They have much in common with each other and with other applied, people-centred professions outside health care such as social work, education, and the advisory and counselling occupational disciplines. There is a common striving among these for professional recognition and for an academically credible knowledge base. All are of a multidisciplinary, practice-based character and are partially founded on bases of knowledge drawn from more 'pure', and therefore higher status, disciplines. Yet all have much to contribute in terms of expertise and excellence in their applied sphere. We should not be afraid, then, of using research methods and theoretical frameworks from a range of disciplines. These will include the physical sciences and medicine, but they will also include the social and behavioural sciences. Social science has much to teach us about diversity of methods and theoretical perspectives. We can also learn a lot from what has already been achieved in social science research. There is no point in reinventing the wheel when we could be pressing on with building the coach and training the horses.

5

The dissemination of research

Beverley French

KEY POINTS

- Dissemination is the transfer of new information, and is influenced by characteristics of the sender, receiver, message and channel of communication
- Two competing perspectives, the instrumental and the transactional, offer different solutions to problems of dissemination
- Evidence for the impact of the three major communication channels – print media, person-to-person contact and the new technologies – are explored in relation to health care
- The current and potential role of publishing, education and the new technologies in dissemination in nursing are considered, together with the role of the public and the impact of the mass media
- Alternative aims for dissemination in the context of decision making in health care are suggested

INTRODUCTION

The process of dissemination (Fig. 5.1) – the transfer of new information from producers to users – would seem to be relatively straightforward. All applied disciplines need ways of transmitting new information to practitioners, and how this can best be done has been a major focus of investigation for the past 30 years. In the earliest studies in agriculture, people were interested in how farmers could be persuaded to use new developments, such as hybrid seed corn, which were disease resistant or had high yields. This type of investigation became known as the study of technology transfer, or *diffusion of innovation*, and rapidly spread to other areas such as engineering, marketing and education (Valente & Rogers 1995). In health care, one of the earliest studies looked at how a new drug diffused into clinical use (Coleman et al 1966). These early studies were mainly concerned with the observational study of passive diffusion: how new developments got transferred into use naturally, without any active efforts to influence practitioners. Later studies began to be interested in how this process could be manipulated to improve uptake.

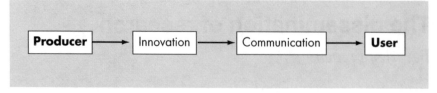

Figure 5.1 Simple represention of linear process of dissemination.

In health care, Lomas & Haynes (1987 p 77) define dissemination as 'the spread of knowledge from its source to health care practitioners. It includes any special efforts to ensure that practitioners acquire a working acquaintance with that knowledge. Successful dissemination therefore requires both accurate communication from the source and accurate understanding by the recipients'.

This definition highlights the roles of both the sender and receiver, emphasising active dissemination rather than reliance on passive diffusion. It also brings attention to 'special efforts' to be undertaken to promote reception of the message by the receiver, and the need for accuracy. Now the simple model of dissemination we started with begins to look a bit more complex (Fig. 5.2).

Is the dissemination of the results of health care research to practitioners successful? The enduring nature of the gap between research findings becoming available and their uptake in clinical practice suggests that things are not as straightforward as might first appear. Even the more com-

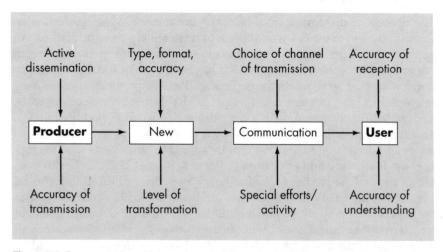

Figure 5.2 Representation of linear process of dissemination with some conditions for success.

Table 5.1   Alternative solutions to the 'problem' of dissemination

	Instrumentalist	Transactional
Problems of communication	Improve quality, increase amount and access	Improve channels, targeting
Problems of reception	Improve skills, provide time and resources	Improve relevance, usefulness, attention to the needs of the user

plex model of dissemination may not be the whole story. Dowie (1996) suggests two competing definitions of what might be the problem:

- a deficiency in communication of results by knowledge producers
- a deficiency in the reception of results by practitioners.

Different perspectives have developed on how to think about this type of problem, and while they might be a little difficult to digest, are worth considering, because they give us different perspectives on what might be a sensible solution (see Table 5.1). The two main viewpoints are the instrumentalist and the transactional.

The instrumentalist view takes as its basis the assumption that the dissemination of relevant information is a rational, linear process. If a practitioner is given information which makes sense and is useful, he or she will use it. It sees practitioners as actively seeking information and motivated to keep abreast, and assumes that they will change their behaviour when they find or are given information that suggests that they ought to.

If problems in dissemination are thought to be caused by deficiencies in the communication of research results by those who produce them, the solution from an instrumentalist viewpoint lies in improving the quality and increasing the availability of disseminated material. One way to do this might be to designate the responsibility for information production to specific agencies, and this solution has been used in action in both the USA and the UK. In 1989 the Public Health Service Act in America was amended to create the Agency for Health Care Policy and Research. The Agency was required by law to create systems to disseminate the results of research and to evaluate the impact of research on the practice of health care. In the UK, the current National Health Service Research and Development (NHS R & D) Information Systems Strategy (ISS) has three major components: the National Research Register, the UK Cochrane Centre; and the NHS Centre for Reviews and Dissemination, specifically aimed at increasing the volume of rigorously created and compiled research-based information and making the information available to the NHS in appropriate formats and media. Chapter 6 discusses these developments.

If problems in dissemination are viewed from the perspective of a deficiency in an audience's ability to receive the message, then methods of influencing audience characteristics or competencies become relevant as a solution, and past and current strategies for dissemination have often focused on this. There is a long history of attempts in nursing to improve uptake of research by guiding practitioners through a structured process of finding and evaluating studies (Horsley et al 1983, Kreuger et al 1978, Stetler & Marram 1976). The current focus on 'evidence-based practice' conceptualises the problem as practitioners' lack of skill in finding, evaluating and using research in practice; a problem which can be improved by a specific type and content of education (Muir Gray 1997).

The transactional model, on the other hand, suggests a more dynamic approach to the relationship between information producers and users. As Huberman (1987 p 589) summarises, 'the gist of this more recent work is roughly that individuals – alone or in organisations – use research in highly selective and strategic ways, ways which might not correspond to what more "instrumentalist" or "utilitarian" theorists might welcome'.

This view focuses much more on the relationships and interactions between knowledge producers and users. Producers are not viewed as impartial, and users are not seen as passive. More attention is paid to:

- motives for producing, disseminating, accessing and using information
- the context in which information uptake occurs
- the consequences of use or non-use.

One explanation for problems from this point of view might concentrate on the fundamental cultural differences between knowledge producers and users, and their political and strategic motives.

From a transactional viewpoint, deficiencies in the communication of research might result from using channels of communication which are inappropriate to practitioners' needs, for example, a reliance on artificial, passive methods of dissemination such as reporting research in journals, or inadequate targeting of the information to relevant users. The transactionalist viewpoint would suggest that the solution would be to pay attention to what kind of information does and does not need to be disseminated, to whom, for what purpose, and what types of transfer might be useful in varying conditions and contexts. This viewpoint might draw attention to the need for local adaptation of national guidelines, or the requirement in some circumstances to transform information into more user-friendly formats. Solutions to this definition of the problem can also be seen in the large scale initiatives in the UK such as the Getting Research into Practice Project (GRiPP), which offers support to groups of practitioners to adapt and use current best evidence to improve care within their own setting.

From a transactional viewpoint, problems in the reception of information by users would be viewed from the assumption of a 'knowledgeable rejecter', rather than the 'ignorant receiver' (Knott & Wildavasky 1980). This view might draw attention to the lack of relevant research, or the irrelevance of much disseminated information to the needs of users, who often want knowledge about new issues that is not available, especially from research. Lack of interest in searching for information might be quite sensible when you know that it is unlikely that you will find an answer to your particular clinical question. Lack of interest in innovative practices by practitioners may also be quite sensible when the information available from the research you *can* find is usually incomplete, untested in the real world, and not relevant to specific settings or patient groups. Solutions that work from this viewpoint might emphasise the involvement of practitioners in research that directly meets their perceived needs, and which is relevant to local contexts. The popularity of action research as a way of involving nurses in the use of research in their local setting is a solution that is more in step with the transactional approach (Clarke et al 1994, Hunt 1987, Lathlean 1989, Pearcey & Draper 1996, White 1984).

These two perspectives, the instrumental and the transactional, do not just apply to dissemination, but are also reflected in what is seen as valid knowledge generally in health care and nursing (see also Chapter 3). Kitson et al (1996) distinguish between the top-down, deductive approach, which suggests that only knowledge that has been rigorously tested should be implemented, and the bottom-up, inductive approach, where more importance is attached to the interpretation of systematic and thorough observation of the current practice context, from which strategies for change can be built. Nursing, especially in the UK, has a strong history of emphasising inductive theory building, and the transactional viewpoint therefore might have its attractions.

However, both viewpoints have their blind spots, and where you are placed on the continuum between research producer and research user might also influence which viewpoint you lean towards. If you are a researcher, you might not want to believe that what you are doing is not relevant or usable, and that it does not attend to the problems of practice, preferring the interpretation that users have not yet received your product, or have not understood it. If you are a practitioner, you might not like to admit that you have failed to attend to relevant material, preferring to believe that it does not exist, or that it is not pertinent to your needs. These competing viewpoints, and your position in the process, might influence what you think would improve the success of dissemination activity.

Taking into consideration these differing perspectives, the rest of the chapter will consider:

- The arguments to support each perspective: the transactional and instrumentalist in relation to dissemination in nursing
- The three major channels available for dissemination: print media;

Table 5.2 Possible explanations and solutions to the 'problem' of dissemination

	Instrumental	Transactional
Deficiency in communication	**Research knowledge does not exist:** *availability of research and systematic review*	**Research does exist, but not in a format that is acceptable to practitioners:** *type, format and transformation of research*
Deficiency in reception	**Research does exist, in acceptable format, but does not reach practitioners:** *skills, resources*	**Research does exist, in acceptable format, but it is not wanted:** *information needs and attitudes to research*

person-to-person contact; and new technologies: the evidence for their impact and their current status

- Potential future developments in dissemination in health care.

THE ARGUMENTS SUPPORTING THE TRANSACTIONAL AND INSTRUMENTALIST PERSPECTIVES

Four competing models for poor dissemination can be postulated. Table 5.2 outlines these and their related explanations (in bold) and solutions (in italics) from the vantage point of the transactional and instrumentalist perspectives. The arguments to support each of these perspectives will be considered in relation to health care generally, and nursing in particular.

Research knowledge doesn't exist

While recent initiatives to increase the volume and quality of disseminated research are impressive, a lack of relevant research may still be a plausible explanation for deficiencies in the transfer of research into practice. In relation to health care, practitioners need to be sure that a set of actions will result in a certain outcome. Research is one type of knowledge which gives practitioners confidence about what will work under certain conditions. Evidence, as in evidence-based practice, appears to refer to knowledge gained from a certain kind of relationship testing in tightly controlled studies. By controlling bias, the proponents of these studies suggest that one may have more confidence that any differences in the results are due to the experimental intervention, not other factors. Using these parameters, it could be argued that in health care we have very little knowledge, and even less evidence. In nursing, we have even less of each, with 80% of the current information for clinical effectiveness relating to medical care (Appelby et al 1995). Nursings' history does not emphasise the specific types of research which recent moves towards increased clinical effectiveness require (i.e. usually controlled trials or at least the use of quantitative methods), and it could be argued that they are not suitable modes of investigation for all nursing problems. However, even including other research designs and taking into account the increase in quality, clinical focus and amount of nursing research (Moody et al 1988), the research is not cumulative. It does not build on previous research, but tends to provide partial answers in lots of different areas (Brown et al 1984). Moreover, it has been predominantly observational (Jacobsen & Meininger 1985), and such designs do not provide strong evidence of cause and effect. Chapters 2 and 3 consider these issues in more detail.

The perceived lack of research has been a common theme in investigations of the barriers to and facilitators of research utilisation in nursing. In one of the first studies, Miller & Messenger (1978) identified the most frequently reported barrier as the lack of relevant research findings available. The WICHE project (see Chapter 1) identified lack of availability of pertinent research as the major barrier to utilisation (Kreuger et al 1978). Funk et al (1989) described several barriers, including lack of relevant research reports. In recent British studies, availability of research in usable formats has been quoted as a major barrier (Lacey 1994, Rogers 1995, Wright 1997).

Against the argument that research does not exist, or does not reach practitioners, MacGuire (1990) and Closs & Cheater (1994) suggest that the opposite may also be true. There may be too much research, leading to information overload, or the information may not be in a format which is accessible to practitioners. MacGuire (1990 p 619) states:

Failure to synthesise means that managers, educators and practitioners are faced with a mass of findings, sometimes conflicting and sometimes based on inadequate research. They do not know what to recommend and may, sensibly, sit tight and do nothing.

Research knowledge does exist, but is not in a format that is acceptable to or usable by practitioners

Kanouse & Jacoby (1988 p 30) contend that summarisation and synthesis of research evidence may not be enough. They suggest that the users' perspective may require different types of information from that found in the research literature and that 'to apply well grounded scientific findings may require making large leaps from the carefully controlled circumstances of the research to the less well controlled circumstances of clinical practice'.

Naylor (1995 p 841) also comments that in view of the limits of the clinical research evidence, 'one might expect paralytic indecisiveness to be more common in practice'. He points out that separate elements in the care of patients which are combined in practice are often tested separately in research studies, providing little valid information on the exact nature of the links between different aspects of care. Thus the outcomes of research are highly dependent on assumptions about one or more poorly defined aspects in the whole model of care. For example, we may know a lot about a single relationship between preoperative preparation and postoperative recovery, but not about how this interacts with the overall quality of care, or the amount of time nurses spend with patients, or the impact of personality, or individual patients' previous experiences of surgery. Nurses often protest that generalisations are not necessarily suitable for individuals, with care decisions having to take into account a host of factors which are not amenable to reduction into discrete, independent components.

The language or jargon of research has consistently been identified as an obstacle to practitioner's understanding (Ludeman 1980). Practitioners complain that research reporting is unnecessarily technical and complicated, that the implications for practice are unclear, and that they do not understand statistical information. Practitioners may find it difficult to transfer findings based on experimental and statistical conclusions to individual practice situations, or to cognitively manage information about uncertainty and risk (Dowie & Elstein 1988). Owen (1995) identifies a difficulty for practitioners who require information that helps them to deal with individual patients, but are faced with the results of research that refers to populations and groups. Tanenbaum (1994), in a small-scale ethnographic study of medical practitioners' use of outcomes research, found that they were primarily reliant on deterministic knowledge: knowledge that is based on the mechanisms of disease and treatment, rather than probabilistic knowledge, which involves knowing about the probability of relationships. Determinism describes the ideal, while probabilism describes the average. Knowing that a particular symptom is present in four out of five people who have a certain disease does not help if you don't know whether your patient is the one person out of five who does not show that symptom. Tanenbaum asserts that while medical practitioners use both types of reasoning, they prefer the anchor of knowledge of the ideal, i.e. trying to understand the mechanisms underlying the disease, rather than predictions based on the average. For this reason, they work through all eventualities, for example, by taking comprehensive histories.

Research knowledge does exist in an acceptable format, but does not reach practitioners

One of the ways in which this argument might be supported is if nurses cannot gain access to the information available. Physical access, to libraries for example, might be problematic. The nursing workforce may have specific requirements for dissemination. Nursing is made up of many specialisms, on multiple, geographically dispersed sites. The centralisation of educational facilities into universities means that libraries are often physically distant from the workplace, and the localisation of trusts means that many cannot support access to large information resources. In Rodgers' (1994) study, some nurses wanted to use library facilities, but were too tired at the end of a shift, or could not gain access at those times.

Even if libraries were accessible, it is not certain that they would provide a major avenue of dissemination for nurses. A number of investigators have studied the reading habits of nurses, and agree that written information is not a preferred source (Fisher & Strank 1971, Haig 1993). Baessler et al (1994), surveying the knowledge sources used by nurses, noted that individual patient data and the nurses' personal experiences were used most commonly. The least commonly used sources were research articles in general and nursing research journals and articles published in medical journals. Vas (1986) studied the reading habits of 344 staff nurses in 10 acute care general hospitals in southern New England. The sample was split between those who reported little or no professional reading, and those who reported reading one or more journals on a regular basis. Similar results were reported in an earlier study of British nurse educators and practitioners (Myco 1980).

In addition to the availability and uptake of resources, it has to be recognised that finding, reading and evaluating research takes time and skill. The lack of time available and practitioners' perceptions of their lack of skill and confidence have been common themes in recent surveys in the UK (Hicks 1996, Pearcey 1995, Rodgers 1994, Veeramah 1995, Wright 1997). However, nurses are not alone in having a lack of skill in evaluating research. Dowie (1996) points out the limitations of an evidence-based approach in medical practice, which does not take into account the analytical inability of doctors. He suggests that unquestioned faith in the decision-making process of the doctor is one of the main reasons for them not undertaking evidence-based practice.

Currently, practitioners faced with explaining the impact of a piece or set of evidence on their decision will usually be found saying that they 'took it into account and bore it in mind', or words to that effect. The precise implications of 'taking into account and bearing in mind' are unknown to most who engage in them and are certainly not explicable to others. The move towards evidence based medicine involves no change in this fundamental fact. (Dowie 1996 p 109)

Further, communication and networking between practitioners, which may serve as a route for sharing and exploring new knowledge between peers, may be severely limited by the intrusion of commercial interests. Information about effective or efficient models of care has potential advantage in the competitive environment of the internal market. The nursing profession has not been characterised by strong collective action in the past (Salvage 1985), and the current emphasis on competition may weaken nursing networks much more than in other professions, who may have stronger inter-organisational contacts. Interest groups run by professional bodies or committed groups of practitioners provide a strong focus for networking, but the sharing of new knowledge may be a secondary consideration to more political or strategic objectives.

Research knowledge does exist in an acceptable format, reaches practitioners, but is not wanted

Information-seeking strategies have been studied extensively in clinical decision making and diagnosis, both in medicine and nursing (Roberts et al 1995), but the role of research-based knowledge is not often specified, and may not be differentiated from other sources of knowledge by practitioners (Luker & Kenrick 1992). Lindblom & Cohen (1979) make the distinction of ordinary knowledge as that which does not come from distinctive professional and social enquiry techniques such as research, but from common sense, thoughtful speculation, or 'casual empiricism' – observing and noting patterns in practice. Rogers (1995) also differentiates between 'software' knowledge (what the innovation is), 'how to' knowledge which details how to use the innovation, and 'principles' knowledge which enlightens the user about how the innovation works (see also Chapter 3).

The practitioner needs information that is specific to his or her setting, and which includes specific 'how to' knowledge, which is not often available in a research reporting format primarily concerned with providing information on validity to the scientific community. Greer (1988) studied the receipt and use of medical information by clinicians in local community hospitals in the USA, the UK and Canada. The practical content of research articles was seen as omitting essential information on the specific procedures, facilities, indications, risks, complications, outliers and outcomes that were necessary for the respondents to judge the degree of similarity with their own individual situations and patients.

It may also be true that practitioners have other needs besides the information content. Smith (1996), in a research review of the clinical information needs of doctors, summarised that these needs were often complex and multidimensional, and included a psychological component of feedback, or support in decision making. Doctors were more likely to seek answers from other doctors, and Smith hypothesised that seeking information from another clinician would better meet the additional psychological need for feedback or support.

Luker & Kenrick (1992) report a small exploratory study which studied what community nurses considered to be the sources of influence on their clinical decisions. The qualitative findings suggested that although the nurses considered that a large proportion of their work required a scientific basis, their practice was largely founded on experiential knowledge, with only three out of 35 influences on clinical decision making originating from research. Another possibility, suggested by Hicks et al (1996), is that the current emphasis on research-based health care results in pressure on health professionals to report a positive orientation to research, while covertly holding negative opinions. Hicks et al used repertory grid technique to elicit how members of a primary health care team construed research and its relationship to their work role. While the results of semi-structured interviews mirrored the usual finding of moderately positive attitudes towards research, repertory grid revealed adverse attitudes, with research not seen to be important or integral to their work role.

As can be seen, there are a number of arguments to support all of the potential viewpoints on whether dissemination is a problem, and if so, why that may be. The next stage is to consider what strategies are available and have been tried in health care and nursing as solutions, and the evidence for their impact.

CHANNELS FOR DISSEMINATION: THE EVIDENCE FOR THEIR IMPACT AND THEIR CURRENT STATUS

There are only a limited number of concrete options for transmitting a message from one person to another. The three main formats or channels of communication that have been studied are:

- the written word or print media
- person-to-person contact
- the new technologies such as electronic transfer, video or computers.

While it may be a simplistic categorisation of the options in a complex process, it helps to set out clearly what the basic options for dissemination are, and their advantages and disadvantages.

Print media

Print media are the major format used in health care for the dissemination of research information, in journals, books, government publications and circulars, monographs, reports and theses. They have the advantage of familiarity, ease of access and relative durability. The disadvantages of reliance on print media are the cost of wide dissemination and the difficulties in adaptation or updating.

Early research demonstrated the ineffectiveness of print media alone in terms of direct utilisation of information (Halpert 1966), and results have continued to be consistent. A recent systematic review (Freemantle et al

1996 p 2) of the effectiveness of printed educational materials in improving the behaviour of health care professionals and patient outcomes concluded 'The effects of printed educational materials compared with no active intervention are at best, small across studies and of uncertain clinical significance'.

A number of studies have empirically tested print media as a method of increasing the awareness and knowledge of nurses. Williams & Roe (1995) used focus groups to evaluate the dissemination of a clinical handbook for continence care to nurses in 15 areas in one health authority (433 nurses were invited to participate, 29% completed the study). Nurses in the control group, who received nothing, significantly improved their knowledge for 59% of the variables. Nurses in the experimental group, who received the handbook, improved their knowledge for 86% of the variables. Luker & Kenrick (1995) studied the impact of a clinical information pack on leg ulcers, designed for attractive information presentation, on the knowledge of 171 community nurses from five districts. The score in the experimental group improved from 26 to 33 out of 62; the score in the control group did not improve. The evidence from these studies suggests that print media have the potential to raise awareness, but that the comparative gains to be made are of questionable clinical significance.

In addition to the provision of print-based research resources, much attention is currently being directed towards transforming raw research into formats that are usable in clinical practice. Clinical guidelines currently represent the major format for communication of research findings to health professionals. Clinical guidelines are systematically developed statements, usually developed by a consensus panel of experts who interpret the available research to make recommendations on the most effective practice. Most of the recent research, in the medical literature especially, has focused on the impact of disseminating consensus recommendations. Direct mailing of consensus recommendations has the capacity to increase awareness (Jacoby & Clark 1986), although the level of awareness may be relatively low. Butler (1986) examined nurses' knowledge of a widely disseminated guideline and found that only 39% of them had received a satisfactory knowledge score. However, the level of awareness can be significantly increased by making the materials visually attractive and/or staging their delivery by dividing them into bite-sized chunks of information (Avorn & Soumerai 1983, Evans et al 1986).

Existing research finds little or no evidence of consensus recommendations leading to action, but demonstrates that they can be successful in some instances. Lomas (1991) suggests that this success may occur when the target audience is already particularly receptive to change and the message is timely and delivered by a credible source in a clinically relevant way. A systematic review of the effect of clinical guidelines on medical practice concluded that they can be effective in influencing practice, if appropriately developed, disseminated and implemented (Effective Health Care 1994). A review of the dissemination and implementation of clinical guidelines in nursing (Cheater & Closs 1997) identified very little evaluative research into methods of guideline dissemination in nursing.

Person-to-person contact

Personal communication is interpreted here in the widest sense as person-to-person communication via the spoken word. This may be one-to-one, or one-to-many, formal or informal, interactive or not. It includes education, conferences, social networking, peer or change agent contact, and academic detailing. The advantages of personal communication for dissemination lie in the opportunity for interaction and feedback, with the potential for adaptation of the message to meet the needs of the user. The main disadvantage is the cost.

In an early research review, Glasser et al (1983) identified the importance of personal communication on knowledge use, including formal and informal contacts, and opportunities for personal communication such as conferences and seminars. Conferences, seminars and workshops were identified as more influential than print media alone. Numerous channels of personal communication for improving the dissemination and uptake of research have been reported in the nursing press, including academic practice collaboration (Mayhew 1994, Verdeber & Urden 1994), networking (Hunt et al 1983) and journal clubs/round tables/interest groups (Kirchoff & Beck 1995, Sheehan 1994, Shortridge-Baggett et al 1994, Tibbles & Sanford 1994), but few have been empirically tested for their effectiveness.

The role and characteristics of the successful change agent and the influence of diffusion networks are major themes in the 'diffusion of innovation' literature which suggests that the practitioners' social network is influential in their uptake of innovation (Rogers 1995). In the medical literature, Keefe et al (1988) suggest that the chance of implementation of research is greater when dissemination is in the local clinical community as opposed to via journals or conferences.

Change agents can be used proactively. Academic detailing is a strategy taken from marketing, which is used extensively by the pharmaceutical companies, and involves personal contact between the clinician and a 'seller'. While this type of role is not common, opinion leaders, change agents or facilitators are increasingly seen in specialist roles in health care: the clinical audit officer, primary care facilitator and clinical nurse specialist are all examples. The clinical nurse specialist as a facilitator of research dissemination and use has been much cited in the nursing literature (Barnard 1986, Collins 1992, Hart et al 1987, Hickey 1990, Huber 1994, Swanson et al 1992), but again its impact has not been evaluated.

New technologies

Despite large-scale developments in the provision of professional education by mass media channels such as television, there is little evidence of their specific use as a means of disseminating research to health care professionals. One exception in the UK was the use of video to disseminate the results of a study on the nursing assessment of patients' pain (Seers & Goodman 1987). In an early and innovative nursing programme in the USA, Barnard & Hoehn (1978) used satellite and telecommunications technology to disseminate knowledge from the Nursing Child Assessment Satellite training project (NCAST) at the University of Washington (see also Chapter 1). The NCAST project was designed to assess the feasibility of using a satellite communications system to disseminate the findings from a major research project to nurses and educators at geographically distant sites. Four communication modes were investigated: two-way communication, one-way communication; video presentation of discussions; and documentation (the control group). Results indicated that groups did not differ significantly in achievement, but that interactive conditions improved confidence and positive attitudes towards the material presented.

The major current influence of technology on research dissemination is via increasing the availability of information. Developments have centred on either the creation of knowledge-based decision support systems, or increasing access to literature. A number of computer systems are available to provide information and assistance with decision making or diagnosis in health care (Henry 1995). One of these has the primary purpose of modelling nursing research knowledge, and is in prototype use at the Virginia Henderson Nursing Library (Graves 1990).

Two current projects are evaluating the impact of improving access for health professionals to databases such as MEDLINE. In America, the National Library of Medicine has funded the RARIN (Retrieval and Application of Research in Nursing) project which aims to experimentally evaluate the installation of computer terminals to health care settings (Bostrom & Wise 1994). In the UK, the recently developed Front-Line Evidence project is evaluating the installation of information searching systems in primary and acute care settings (Donald 1996).

In summary, the major channels of transmission of research in current use in health care all have inherent features which influence their reception, uptake and use by practitioners. The evidence suggests that print media have the potential to influence awareness, but that personal contact has the capacity to be more influential in terms of the receptivity and behaviour of the user. The jury is still out on the impact of the newer forms of technology: evidence on the impact of their use is as yet limited in health care. The next three sections will consider the current status of these major channels for dissemination.

Print media: problems with publishing in nursing

Print media, mainly in the form of books and journals, remain the major source of information for most professional groups. Publishers can be seen as 'knowledge brokers' in professional practice, acting as translators and interpreters between the research community and practitioners. They play a valuable role in encouraging new authors, highlighting trends, responding to practice needs, formalising the system for linking people and information, unifying fields of knowledge, and validating research. They work with a prescribed format for communication which is international and universally accepted.

Journals particularly, with their known conventions for reporting and reviewing content, provide practitioners with a source which can itself be evaluated and trusted. In common with other professional groups, journal sources for nursing are increasing rapidly. There are hundreds of journals directed at different segments of the profession, some focusing on content interest, such as health care computing or quality assurance, and others on specialist areas of clinical practice, such as intensive care or community nursing. These journals can be divided into those whose main function is to provide educational, clinical and news information for practitioners on general current issues, and those whose main function is to maintain communication between researchers, and, through peer review, to evaluate and validate research and research conclusions. However, this distinction is becoming less valid, with most professional journals now reporting some research. A review of the research content of 12 major nursing journals between 1975 and 1985 found that the research content increased from 14% in 1975 to 22% in 1985 (Kilby et al 1991). A recent development has been the research review journal, such as *Journal of Clinical Effectiveness* and *Evidence-Based Nursing*, which aim to provide standardised summaries and evaluations of good-quality research. While this new hybrid is clearly targeted at practitioners, not researchers, it is a generic publication for the profession, and is not targeted at a specific segment. For this reason, it remains to be seen whether such journals will be directly accessed by practitioners.

The problem with publishing in nursing, as in any professional group, lies in the limitations of the media, and contradictions in its purpose. The accepted format for research reporting has the purpose of making public the essential details of the method by which the information was created, so that its validity can be evaluated by other researchers and reviewers. The format is not designed to communicate to practitioners the implications of the research for their practice. The purpose of publication is associated with its role in the scientific process of communication, and the evaluation of research quality. This is evidenced by the use of criteria related to the assessment of research publications in the Research Assessment Exercise (RAE) (Box 5.1) (see also Chapter 3).

Box 5.1 The Research Assessment Exercise (RAE)

The Research Assessment Exercise (RAE), conducted every 4 years across universities and academic subjects, is a public report of the assessment of the quality of research in universities in the UK. Assessment is based on such criteria as the number of post-graduate students, research grants awarded and research publications, with reward for excellence a key feature. The RAE is very influential because funding decisions for research are based on the results.

The RAE places heavy pressure on academics to publish, and there may be a strong incentive to publish innovative material or positive results, possibly prematurely. Against the strong rationale for publishing the results of nursing research in the professional journals, the RAE gives more weight to publications in scholarly journals (Tierney 1994), with the consequence that those journals perceived to be of high scientific merit are overloaded. While this may not in itself be a bad thing, the impact on the dissemination of current research is quite severe. Material submitted to one publisher cannot be submitted elsewhere, and remains in limbo until a decision is made about whether it will be accepted, which can take many months, even years. In the process of publication, copyright is signed over to the publisher, and while this clearly acts to protect both the rights of the author and the commercial rights of the publisher, it limits the free dissemination of the results of research. Although researchers have always published their work in different journals to disseminate their work to different audiences, there is now perhaps more temptation to fragment reporting, not for different audiences, but for different publication opportunities to improve their RAE rating (Box 3.3 summarises the impact values of various journals). In addition, the international nature of some journals means that some of their contents may not relate to nursing practice in this country.

Publishers also prefer research that reports positive results. Good news is attractive to the audience; the 'Journal of Negative Results and Failed Ideas' is not likely to sell well. This means that high-quality research which finds that an innovation in some aspect of nursing care is not any more effective than current practice is less likely to be published than other studies which report that the innovation is more effective. As a consequence, our view of the efficacy of an innovation is biased by the bias in publication towards 'positive' results. Leaving aside the potential for data falsification in research for other reasons (Resnik 1996), this publication bias may increase the pressure on researchers to report positive results which are not entirely justified by the data. Journals can also be a source of resistance to new ideas, with the peer review system prone to conceptual inbreeding (Campanario 1995) whereby the system acts to protect established researchers' vested interests by controlling entry to publication. It would be difficult to say whether publishers act as referees or censors, but they clearly have a gate-keeping role on what is classed as acceptable knowledge.

Although the number of textbooks has quadrupled in the last decade (Kilby et al 1989), they take even longer from conception to publication. Textbooks were ranked higher than journals in nurses' preferred sources of information (Corcoran-Perry & Graves 1990). They appear more authoritative, but have been found to be seriously deficient in reporting the latest findings from research (Antman et al 1992). Textbooks generally cover a whole field, are relatively expensive, and quickly become outdated. However, they are a major source of information, especially in pre-qualifying training.

While research in books and journals appear on first examination to be an instrumentalist tool, the motives for and strategic uses of publication can also be seen from a transactionalist view. Researchers, whose survival is dependent on the RAE, are unlikely to selflessly lay down personal interests and spend time transforming their research if this disadvantages them, despite wholehearted agreement that this should be their primary purpose.

Personal contact: the impact of continuing education

The requirements of the Post Registration Education and Practice Project (PREPP) reinforce the responsibility of the individual practitioner to maintain and develop professional knowledge and competence (United Kingdom Central Council for Nursing, Midwifery and Health Visiting 1992). Project 2000, with its emphasis on the nurse as a knowledgeable doer, has done much to promote the concept of everyday professional practice being based on systematic scientific enquiry. Research methodology and critical appraisal are increasingly a component of pre-qualifying and post-basic education.

The Task Force for the Strategy for Research in Nursing, Midwifery and Health Visiting (Department of Health 1993a) outlined a structure for research within the nursing profession, based on a foundation of awareness and understanding of research amongst the profession as a whole, with a smaller number of practitioners progressing to the advanced skills required to undertake research. To date, the main method of teaching research in pre- and post-basic nursing education has been based on gaining skills by participation in the research process, with an implicit value placed on creating new knowledge. Emphasis on the requirement for rigour in the process of creating new knowledge has been assumed to lead to skill and rigour in the process of using research information created by others. Courses specifically aimed at research appraisal and utilisation therefore have not been widely available. A survey of the research content of American master's degree programmes found that only 14% included content on the research utilisation process (Firlit et al 1987). This appears to be changing, and there have been a number of recent reports of courses in research utilisation in nursing (Floyd 1996, Lacey 1996, Miller 1996, Pond & Bradshaw 1996, Spence-Lazinger et al 1993).

The content of educational courses in research utilisation in nursing tend to concentrate on the validity and reliability of research methods. A new approach, principally developed at McMaster University in Canada, is to use the principles of clinical epidemiology to consider the research evidence for a clinical question relating to an individual patient or client. This method concentrates firstly on the type of research design necessary to provide a valid answer to a question of therapeutic effectiveness, or assessment, or risk, before considering effective search strategies and appraisal of study quality. This approach encourages the practitioner to focus on a specific question and target relevant high-quality research to reduce the amount of redundant material that needs to be sifted through. However, it relies heavily on the practitioner's ability to access multiple information sources – usually databases held on compact disc in libraries – and to perform keyword searches of the literature (Mulhall 1996).

Many practitioners are familiar with these sources, but they may not be skilled in their use. A number of recent initiatives in the UK aim to teach the skills of critical appraisal using epidemiological principles, relying mainly on systematic review as the most likely source of rigorous information for practitioners. These initiatives might include an introduction to sources of systematic review such as The Cochrane Library, but do not usually teach search skills, although some agencies, for example, North Thames Research Appraisal Group are planning or offer such courses. Education directed at teaching medical students how to ask appropriate clinical questions, perform targeted searches, appraise the results and apply them in practice has demonstrated enduring effects in one study (Shin et al 1993). Clinicians who had been taught this method in basic training were more likely to maintain up-to-date knowledge of advances in treatment.

Continuing education might also impact on the dissemination of research in more diffuse ways, by encouraging practitioners to access and use literature more frequently, by promoting a more positive approach to research, or by highlighting research, which then influences the practitioners' awareness and behaviour (Haines & Jones 1994). Reviews of the impact of continuing education identify gains in knowledge, some evidence for behavioural change, but little impact on the clinical outcome of care (Barriball et al 1992, Bayley 1988, Warmuth 1987). A systematic review of the effectiveness of continuing medical education in changing practice demonstrated that approaches that relied solely on giving information were not successful in promoting behavioural change. Approaches that included facilitating the desired change in the practice site, or reinforcers by reminder or feedback, were more likely to be successful than those which relied solely on communicating or disseminating information

(Davies et al 1995). One nursing study (Linde 1989) experimentally tested the impact of education on the degree of research use in nursing. Linde (1989) tested three levels of communication about a practice innovation on attitudes to utilisation and propensity to change. The provision of written information and the provision of education in addition to written information produced a significant increase in utilisation and the propensity to change.

Common sense would suggest that the provision of experience or education in research or its utilisation would increase the potential for dissemination and use in practice. However, to date, hard evidence of impact on clinical outcome is lacking. Chapman (1996) identifies the potential costs to both the individual and the organisation of continuing education and training. Staff replacement, library facilities, access to computers, personal time and financial costs for travel all need to be funded. While the need for continuing education may appear to be self-evident, justification for the associated costs in the light of the lack of evidence of impact on clinical outcomes is difficult in an era of fiscal restraint. Other less costly methods may be seen as more appropriate.

Use of mass media for dissemination, and the role of the public

The reviews of Glasser et al (1983) and Rogers (1995) suggest that mass media influence awareness, but do not influence the amount or timing of uptake of innovation. Newspapers, magazines, radio, video and television have not to date been widely used to disseminate research information to health professionals. Their advantages – wide coverage, generic appeal, timeliness and ease of access – are also their weaknesses: the difficulty in targeting specific audience segments, the cost of production for a one-off audience, and the continual updating that would be required. Dedicated mass media channels, such as television programmes broadcast at times designed for videoing, are becoming more popular, but in the near future it is more likely that mass media campaigns will alter professional practice patterns through changing the perceptions and behaviour of the public.

The people with the most to gain from effective health care are the patients, and informing patients can help them to influence the care they receive and improve the outcome (Greenfield et al 1985). Hope (1996) describes current projects in the UK centred on evidence-based patient choice, and Entwistle et al (1996) provide a clear summary of evidence-based practice for people working in areas responsible for providing health care information to the public. The mass media are also being used to provide health care data to the public on the performance of health care organisations. Benton (1997) reports on one example in the USA, the Greater Cleveland Health Quality Choice Coalition, a project which publishes performance data in the form of patient outcome and satisfaction data on a wide range of hospitals across a range of common medical, surgical and obstetric conditions. The information is adjusted to take account of different case mix, and so provides a fair comparison, and is widely reported in the media. Despite recent attempts to provide comparative information on health service performance on indicators of quality such as the Patient's Charter, the UK lags well behind the USA in this respect. A recent White Paper, *The National Health Service: A Service with Ambitions* (Department of Health 1996c) identifies information as an area for action, with the provision of information to users as a key method of empowering users to make informed decisions about their own care.

New technologies such as multimedia are being used to present research-based treatment decision options to patients (Eve 1995), and have been shown to influence their preference for specific treatments. In one study, the provision of information to patients on the treatment options for prostate disease markedly influenced the uptake of various treatment options (Agency for Health Care Policy and Research 1995). These new technologies are beginning to be used to provide patient information in the UK; for example, Nottingham University is creating a multimedia package specifically aimed at helping children to participate in decisions about how they are treated for enuresis (Morris 1996).

The most common use of the mass media is to front a 'total dissemination push', predominantly aimed at the public on major topical health issues, such as drug abuse. The mass media have been used successfully to communicate the results of health care research to both the general public and professionals. A recent example is the media push to advertise changes to babies' sleeping positions to prevent sudden infant death syndrome (Scott et al 1994). However, the public are increasingly seeking out health and science news for themselves, this interest being reflected by the fact that many newspapers and magazines contain a regular health care section. The major weakness with the use of mass media for dissemination of research findings to the public is that the reporting tends to be superficial, with insufficient detail for the public to apply the results to their own lives, and simplification which results in inaccurate information (Ankney et al 1996).

POTENTIAL FUTURE DEVELOPMENTS
Innovative methods of dissemination

Overall, the evidence suggests that mechanisms to improve uptake of research are available and can be successful, but that 'effective dissemination will depend on using multiple means to communicate key messages rather than a single measure or "magic bullet"'(Freemantle & Watt 1994 p 133).

Methods which might improve dissemination include strategies to:

- increase access
- alter presentation
- target users
- increase natural diffusion.

Increasing access

Current dissemination methods rely heavily on the organisational structures in place in provider units. New clinical effectiveness information is flagged in Executive Letters (ELs) from the NHS Executive to chief executives of trusts, who are sent copies of all new systematic reviews and reports. Organisations will have a mechanism in place to circulate the information to appropriate personnel, usually through the management hierarchy. Copies are then stored in a library or resource facility. Reliance on a few copies of reports circulating through an organisation with perhaps 1000 nurses is clearly not adequate. In my own experience, practising nurses are often not aware of current information, or the existence of the EL telling them what is available.

The NHSnet (Box 5.2) may be a solution to the problems of managing communication and dissemination of research in such a large organisation. The Internet is rapidly becoming an alternative information source for professionals and the public (Laporte 1994), and despite the difficulty with sifting the good information from the not so good, it offers huge potential for the rapid and effective dissemination of research-based knowledge, bypassing most of the potential problems of access to print-based media. Most of the existing evidence-based practice resources such as the Cochrane Collaboration and the NHS Centre for Reviews and Dissemination have a site on the Internet (Booth 1996). Most journals will also be electronically accessible, but they will be markedly different from current print versions. The electronic journal of the future will include articles with video, audio or multimedia presentations, with automatic links to other sources that open if selected.

Box 5.2 The NHSnet

The NHSnet is a computer-based communication network which will link up all health facilities in the UK, providing access to a messaging service, an NHS directory, and an Internet service for use within the NHS.

Matthews (1995) envisages the impact of the Internet on publishing. Instead of the current peer review system, articles would be posted on the

NET and comment allowed; authors could then submit revised versions of their work, although the original would remain. Articles would then become living documents, and the time delay for publishing would be bypassed. Protagonists argue that abolishment of the peer review system as it stands would reduce the quality of material to the level of current entries to bulletin boards on the NET. Matthews suggests that a future system could safeguard quality by charging authors to publish in refereed electronic journals, which are cheaper to produce than paper-based formats, rather than charging subscriptions to readers. This may be good for the individual nurse who has computer access and skills, but may be bad for the nursing profession if it reduces the opportunities for practitioners to publish.

Computer systems are also improving the selection and targeting of information to the appropriate audience. Updating information services are available in which the user can signify preferences for information on specific topics, and which will search out that information and inform the user of its availability. Computerised reminder systems are being used to bring relevant research findings to the notice of the professional at the point of decision making, for example, prescribing, or ordering diagnostic tests. Intelligent decision support systems are being combined with knowledge databases to compute the risks and benefits of alternative decisions tailored to individual patients, and also to provide knowledge-based systems which incorporate current standardised guidelines at the point and time of decision making and delivery of patient care (Gordon 1995). For example, the current guidelines for management of paediatric asthma would be available on a computer screen as the general practitioner is prescribing, or in the accident and emergency department.

Altering presentation

The principles of marketing, which are based on finding out the needs of target markets and satisfying them, have not been used to any great degree in the dissemination of health care information, despite the success of drug companies in influencing professional behaviour. Marketing principles are beginning to influence the more comprehensive dissemination and utilisation strategies such as GRiPP, counterbalancing the top-down approach of most dissemination initiatives (Dickinson 1995). The use of commercial methods of presentation, such as including illustrations and a familiar format for content, has been used for dissemination activity in nursing (Luker & Kenrick 1995).

A field of development which has been largely ignored is the use of novel methods of presentation for complex information. Their potential is being recognised in other fields, for example city guides (Wurman 1991). Knowledge in health care can be contained and represented as the relationships between variables, and complex quantitative information such as that contained in multiple research studies can be visually displayed by using diagrams. This allows the user to visualise the information as a whole, rather than as a series of discrete bits of data. The capacity of the new computer-based technologies to use three-dimensional graphic or moving representation has hardly impacted at all on the transmission and transformation of complex information from research. Imagine being able to see research results unfold visually, with tables and graphs slowly building, illustrating differences between, say, the experimental and control groups in a randomised controlled trial.

Interactive multimedia is a compact or laser disc-based technology which allows large volumes of audio, video, graphic and print media to be programmed into a learning experience. Interactivity refers to the amount of interaction between the needs and interests of the individual user and the programme, provided by options such as speed and sequencing of presentation or selectivity of content. Levels of interactivity vary, dependent on the programming, but the sophistication of children's video games gives an insight into the capability of these programmes. Interactive multimedia has been found to be effective in relation to recall of material in comparison with lectures or demonstrations (Schare et al 1991). The technology is used in nursing education (Lyte & Kershaw 1994), and is beginning to be used for the provision of patient information, but has not yet been widely used to improve the presentation of research information for professionals.

Targeting users

The latest communications approaches are moving away from the linear 'product push' instrumentalist view, towards an acknowledgement of the transactionalist view that research uptake is governed by social structures that are locally constructed and context-specific (Dawson 1995). Many nurses look to their professional association for research information. Supporting the common interests of group members and fostering their interaction results in information exchange. Personal contact between peers, or exposure to the views of a respected opinion leader, have been shown to be influential in determining whether an innovation will be tried (Glasser et al 1983, Rogers 1995). The social context of research dissemination and use is being increasingly recognised in current UK projects. The evaluation of the Framework for Appropriate Care Throughout Sheffield (FACTS) project suggests that the source of the message is clearly influential in decisions made by practitioners. Participants have been influenced to join the project by the number of other people involved, and by having the opportunity to gain information from a variety of sources (Musson 1996). Similarly, the Promoting Action on Clinical Effectiveness (PACE) programme (Dunning & Cooper 1996) provides local networks with support and funding to develop and implement specific research-based service developments.

Improving personal contact does not have to be limited to local contexts. Specialist groups in nursing particularly would benefit from methods of increasing personal communication, without the need to travel large distances. Dissemination of information in existing networks has perhaps placed too much reliance on print media alone, and one possibility is to record network meetings or conferences for wider distribution. Sigma Theta Tau, a nursing society in the USA, videotapes its conferences (Butts 1982), and audiotapes of other conferences are often also available (e.g. The Scientific Basis of Health Services Conference 1995). The NHS network will include an e-mail facility, allowing fast, text-based communication between people in distant sites, and will also in time allow the delivery and transmission of more complex material such as video. Real-time digital transmission of video is currently used in conferencing people in geographically distant sites, such as virtual surgeries for consultants and virtual classrooms for students. This type of communication could stimulate natural dissemination by improving communication between peers, or by providing an interactive facility for communication between researchers and users who are geographically distant.

Altering direction of dissemination

An alternative view of dissemination is to increase the amount of information which is available from clinical practice. Developments in technology have created the possibility of collating large datasets which, because of their size, can be used to identify variation, and process–outcome relationships. The TELENURSING programme is a European Union funded project to promote the collection of a standard minimum dataset of clinical nursing information, which would be collected on each patient, to provide collatable and comparable data on the problems, interventions and outcomes of nursing (Mortensen & Nielsen 1995).

The attraction of large datasets of information on nursing outcomes is easy to see. Collecting a minimum amount of data from each episode of patient care would allow comparison of outcomes across settings. If one site had better outcomes despite similarities in case mix and resource input, the reasons could be investigated and best practice shared. The collection and ownership of information that has been created from practice allows the bottom-up development of a research agenda, which is grounded in the intrinsic motivation of a profession to improve practice. The disadvantages of these developments lie in the danger that the description of nursing will be simplified into discrete, concrete tasks which can be easily coded, echoing the problems of current workload classification systems.

These developments identify the major transformations in dissemination that are slowly taking place and can be summarised as from:

- paper to electronic media
- informatics to telematics
- professional to public information.

If you have recently spent many futile hours trying to obtain a report that you have heard about, which you thought might contain useful information for your job, and you have not been able to trace it, cannot afford to buy it, or are unable to get to a library to borrow it, you would be forgiven for thinking that these developments seem a long way off. However, before they are dismissed, consider the example of how education is developing.

The virtual university: a view of the future?

Conventional learning requires the individual to attend a specific institution. Distance learning courses presently allow people to study up to higher degree level, even if they live in communities that are geographically isolated, or if they work in jobs that make regular attendance at an educational institution difficult. The most successful institution for distance learning in the UK has been the Open University, which provides a huge range of courses, supported by high-quality learning materials and radio and television programmes.

As commuter travel becomes more difficult, and people become more familiar with accessing different forms of technology, education is becoming much more flexible in how it is delivered and accessed (Davidson & Rhodes 1996). Students can access some courses from their computers at home or at work, and participate in discussion with other students and lecturers via e-mail and bulletin boards. Assignments, course notes and even course textbooks can be sent and delivered electronically. Course materials can include video, graphic and sound clips. The advantages are obvious. Courses can be taken at any time, and course materials can be rapidly updated to include the latest research, with new materials tagged so that students can revisit the course and update their knowledge. The cost to the user in telephone connection time is likely to be outweighed by savings in the cost of travel.

This level of development may seem futuristic, but the reality is that most of these components are in use now. Video communications technology for interactive distance learning has been tested within nurse education in the UK (Emery 1996). A virtual library is operational in the Genesis Project in Cumbria (Hendry 1997). In my own institution at the University of Central Lancashire, students on remote sites access library services online, interactive multimedia programmes are used for science teaching in all nursing programmes, and I have been involved in a prototype multi-media development for teaching a specific aspect of nursing care, which incorporates the research literature. This type of resource illustrates how the best currently available evidence for effective clinical practice can underpin educational programmes in nursing practice.

CD-ROM technology is set to revolutionise higher and professional education. Interactive media is affordable to a mass audience, can meet the flexible delivery requirements of a large workforce with 24-hour cover, and is particularly suited to delivery on geographically dispersed sites. The major aim of the project was to link the research evidence for best practice into a learning resource in the form of an illustrated guideline for care. Using multimedia allowed us to incorporate video clips of related nursing procedures, and photographs of equipment, alongside abstracts of related research at any point in the programme. The research base is designed to be comprehensive, and prototype development aims to use visual methods of presentation for complex concepts, and to include video footage of the major researchers for each topic.

The prototype is intended primarily for personal computer use in provider units or in educational institutions, either as an encyclopaedic resource that practitioners can interrogate to question the research base relevant to specific practice, or as a planned learning experience. The specific advantages of multimedia technology in relation to dissemination of research in health care are the facilitation of:

- Novel techniques for presenting and explaining research including the use of video, animation, textual and graphic modes to illustrate complex information such as relationships, perspective, context or development over time.
- User choice, control and flexibility over the direction, depth and pace of presentation, adapting the presentation of research information to the needs of different audiences, for example novice or expert practitioners.
- Continuous updating, and the incorporation of new evidence.

Impact of new technology on dissemination

The advantages of new technologies for dissemination are easily identified. New technologies such as CD-ROM facilitate the production, storage and transfer of large volumes of information. Information transfer is fast, and can easily incorporate new media. They are cheap to replicate, and can be accessed by multiple users simultaneously. They reduce the handicap of geographical distance and, in theory, are not dependent on expensive human expertise. The disadvantages of new technologies include the high cost of development and production, with large initial capital costs in accessing systems, such as the purchase of computers. Computer technology develops rapidly and is quickly redundant, and in practice is heavily dependent on expensive human technical expertise. However, costs reduce relative to the number of people who have access, and computers are not supposed to have bad days.

CONCLUSION

The hidden consequences of technological development on dissemination are not with the technology itself, but in the use that humans make of it. Ultimately, it depends on what we are aiming for. Are we aiming:

- To disseminate knowledge or information? Technology improves the storage of information, but does not of itself improve its quality, and there is the real possibility of increasing the volume of available information with no increase in the quality of knowledge.
- For transmission, or transformation? Technology increases opportunities for transmission, and there are great possibilities for technology to be utilised in the transformation of information, but these are to date largely unexplored in relation to the transformation of research into formats acceptable to practitioners.
- For top-down or bottom-up communication? There is a tendency to think of dissemination as one way traffic, from the knowledge producers to the knowledge users, but technology could provide the tools for the routine collation of data, empowering the development of knowledge grounded in the realities of everyday practice.
- To inform, to coerce or to control? Technology of itself does not appear to coerce, but ownership of information allows control by comparison, identification of variance, and assignment of responsibility for the outcomes of care. At a more sinister level, access to computerised sites can be monitored, potentially allowing the identification of those who have and those who have not accessed information. Records of access may, and probably will be used in the social marketing of research, if not in the identification of individuals.

In summary, technology is here to stay, and as with other strategies can be used for good or evil in whichever model of dissemination is subscribed to. There is a complex set of issues surrounding the implementation of research. Current strategies are predominantly influenced by the dominance of the instrumentalist paradigm, and motivated by a vision that there are research resources that are under-utilised which, if tapped, could benefit patient care. This apparently simple purpose, to move information from those who have it to those who do not, and the assumption that practitioners will change their practice as a result of research is increasingly being questioned. Transactional models emphasise the role of dissemination in power relationships, and the potential use of dissemination as a coercive strategy. Before we can design strategies to improve the use of research, perhaps we need to pay more attention to understanding the role that dissemination plays in decision making in the context of health care (Dopson et al 1994).

6

Using research and the role of systematic reviews of the literature

Nicky Cullum Jacqueline Droogan

KEY POINTS

- Research should be made relevant and accessible to practitioners
- Systems should be put in place to help practitioners make sense of the large volume of research in health care
- Literature searching and critical appraisal are skills which need to be learned
- Systematic reviews locate, appraise and synthesise the body of research on a particular topic to obtain a reliable overview; they are essential reading when keeping abreast of research
- The Cochrane Library, which incorporates the Cochrane Database of Systematic Reviews and the Database of Abstracts of Reviews of Effectiveness (DARE), is the primary source of high-quality systematic reviews of health care
- The Practice and Service Development Initiative based at the National Health Service Centre for Reviews and Dissemination (NHS CRD), University of York, UK, has developed a model of disseminating high-quality systematic reviews to change agents in nursing and the therapy professions

INTRODUCTION

Briggs (1972) recommended that nursing become a research-based profession; however, the journey has been difficult and we have not yet arrived! For some, caring is what nursing is all about, and caring is not up for evaluation (in the sense of an experiment). We would argue that whilst caring and respect for others should be at the heart of all that nurses do, strategies for palliation and cure must also be evaluated.

There are innumerable clinical situations where nurses must make informed clinical decisions between alternative ways of doing things. For example:

- what type of mattress or bed should we provide for a patient who is at risk of a pressure sore?
- how do we prevent infection in a patient who has an indwelling urethral catheter?
- how should we support new mothers who want to breast feed?
- how might we reduce the rates of accident in children and adolescents?
- what types of support do women with breast cancer benefit from?

Such decisions might be about individual patients and clients, whole communities, or the organisation of services, and need to be informed by the appropriate body of research. Patients expect nurses to be caring, but they also expect that the things that nurses 'do' are tried and tested.

So many journals – so little time

To deliver research-based care, it goes without saying that we need to be 'on top of' the research, but no individual can do this without considerable help. Internationally there are 499 journals about nurses and nursing (Ulrich's International Periodicals Directory 1996) and thousands of research articles highly relevant to nurses which are published in other health, medical, psychological, sociological and educational journals. Unfortunately, nurses, midwives and health visitors are frequently battling against an ever-increasing workload, and even if they are afforded the necessary time, they often do not have access to the journals they need (Meah et al 1996, Moorbath 1996). Also, most of us are unable to understand papers written in languages other than our own, and are therefore likely to miss valuable research. Of course, even if we access research we do not necessarily use it. Bostrom & Suter (1993) reported that only 23% of 1588 practising nurses thought that they had made a change in practice based on research during their career. Similarly, Luker & Kenrick (1995) found that community nurses were aware of research, but did not perceive it as informing their practice.

Sorting out the wheat from the chaff

Where is the knowledge we have lost in information?

(T. S. Eliot, *The Rock*, part 1)

As anyone who has searched the literature seeking a quick answer to an apparently simple question knows, there is only a small amount of high-quality nursing research with relevance for practice out there, and it is difficult to find. The easiest, but most biased way of finding the answer to a clinical question is to quickly scan through the journals that you happen to have on your shelves. You are quite likely to find something of relevance if your question concerns an everyday topic. However, it might take you a long time to find it and you will not necessarily know how the one or two papers that you locate compare with the total body of research in that area. This is particularly important to know if you are trying to ascertain 'best practice'. If you have access to a library, you could use one of the electronic bibliographical databases that routinely abstract and index papers published in the international literature (see Box 6.1). MEDLINE (produced by the National Library of Medicine in the USA) indexes approximately 3700 journals from 1966 onwards, whilst CINAHL (the Cumulative Index of Nursing and Allied Health Literature) is primarily concerned with nursing and the therapies. Interestingly, a recent comparison of these two databases found MEDLINE to be a more fruitful source of references related to specific nursing topics (Brazier & Begley 1996).

Literature searching is a skill, and librarians are there to help us develop this skill. The best searches of electronic bibliographical databases use a combination of the Subject Headings (in MEDLINE these are called MeSH terms – indexing tags or keywords determined by the database and attributed to each paper by trained indexers), and free text. MeSH terms are accessed via the Thesaurus function of MEDLINE and it is important to try and use every synonym for the subject in question. When you use a textword to search for papers, you avoid relying on the indexers, but you do rely on the author of the paper using that word. For example, a search for randomised controlled trials in nursing found that reference to the term 'randomised controlled trial' was often missing from titles and abstracts, resulting in many studies being missed by a MEDLINE search (Cullum 1997). There are three important ways of saving time and improving the reliability of the information that you seek through electronic searching:

1. first, look for reliable summaries of research on the topic on interest, i.e. systematic reviews (see below)
2. if the systematic reviews are older than 1 year, or you are unable to find one, look for research articles
3. use the appropriateness of the research design to filter the wheat from the chaff: go for the *best available* evidence.

Systematic reviews are where the reviewer strives to:

- identify and obtain *all* the research on a topic
- minimise bias in the analysis and interpretation of the original research.

By searching for systematic reviews as a priority, you will reduce the likelihood of being influenced by a biased sample of the literature and you will save much time, as the primary research (i.e. those articles which make up the review) will already have been appraised and synthesised by the reviewer.

When looking at primary research, filtering by research design enables

---

Box 6.1   Bibliographic databases

MEDLINE
The National Library of Medicine's bibliographic database. It is one of the major sources for biomedical information. MEDLINE corresponds to three printed indexes: Index Medicus; the Index to Dental Literature; and the Index to Nursing Literature. Approximately 400 000 records are added each year.

CINAHL (Cumulative Index to Nursing and Allied Health Literature)
This database is designed to meet the information needs of nurses and allied health professionals. It provides access to virtually all English-language nursing journals, publications from the American Nurses' Association and the National League for Nursing, and primary articles from 13 allied health journals.

AMED (Allied and Alternative Medicine)
A bibliographic database covering the fields of complementary or alternative medicine. AMED is produced by the British Library.

English National Board Health Care Database
A database of over 25 000 references from the major nursing journals, research and report references, open learning packages and programmes, and details of relevant organisations.

BIDS (Bath Information and Data Services)
The ISI citations indexes contained on BIDS are bibliographic indexes covering scientific and technical information, social sciences, arts and humanities. Data are taken from about 7500 selected international journals from 1981 onwards.

ASSIA (Applied Social Sciences Index and Abstracts)
ASSIA provides a comprehensive reference service on modern society and its problems. Aspects of law, business, national politics and, in particular, local government are included. It has a strong emphasis on the applied aspects of the social sciences.

EMBASE (Excerpta Medica)
Current and comprehensive pharmacological and biomedical database. It concentrates on European sources, and is renowned for its coverage of the drug-related literature. It consists of abstracts and citations to over 3500 journals published in 110 countries.

PsychLIT
Database of the American Psychological Association. Contains references and some abstracts to journal articles and books. Updated quarterly.

---

you to discard those studies which are likely to provide biased, unreliable answers. Quite what the best available evidence looks like depends on the question. If your question is one of effectiveness (as are those listed earlier), then a well-conducted randomised controlled trial (RCT) is the design of choice – it is least susceptible to bias and overestimation of the effect of the intervention in question (Muir Gray 1997). However, if you are looking for a deeper understanding of how people with a particular condition, say AIDS, might feel about their diagnosis, then you would seek qualitative designs such as phenomenology, and an RCT would be wholly inappropriate (see also Chapter 3 for a discussion of 'evidence'). Hierarchies of evidence have been designed for studies investigating cause and effect relationships (see Box 6.2; other examples include Elwood 1988, Woolf et al 1990). These hierarchies are grounded in the notion that some study designs protect against bias better than others. The higher up the hierarchy a study is, the more confidently we can attribute outcome effects to the particular intervention and not to other factors. It should be emphasised that such hierarchies are only intended to describe cause and effect relationships and do not suggest that quantitative research is better than qualitative, as has been suggested by some (Hicks & Hennessy 1997).

Box 6.2   An example of a hierarchy of evidence

| I | Well-designed randomised controlled trial |
| | Other types of trial |

II–1a	Well-designed controlled trial with pseudo-randomisation
II–1b	Well-designed controlled trial with no randomisation
	Cohort study
II–2a	Well-designed cohort (prospective study) with concurrent controls
II–2b	Well-designed cohort (prospective study) with historical controls
II–2c	Well-designed cohort (retrospective study) with concurrent controls
II–3	Well-designed case-control (retrospective) study

| III | Large differences from comparisons between times and/or places with and without intervention (in some circumstances these may be equivalent to level II or I) |

| IV | Opinions of respected authorities based on clinical experience: descriptive studies and reports of expert committees |

NHS Centre for Reviews and Dissemination (1996)

Appraising original research

The crunch comes once a research report has been located: can the findings be trusted? Are they worthy enough to change practice? This is where critical appraisal comes in. It is our personal perception that for too long nurses have been taught how to *do* research, but have been insufficiently prepared for the appraisal of research that has been completed by others. Appraisal checklists do appear in nursing texts, but they tend to focus on reporting style (e.g. Is the title of the paper appropriate? Are the aims of the research clear?) rather than whether the research methods were appropriate to the question, and the likely validity and reliability of the findings. A number of excellent texts about critical appraisal are published elsewhere (e.g. Sackett et al 1991, 1997) and the series by the Evidence Based Medicine Working Group published in the *Journal of the American Medical Association* (1993–1996) is available on the World Wide Web [http://hiru.mcmaster.ca/ebm/userguid/].

RCTs (sometimes called experimental studies) have often been undertaken to explore the effectiveness of different nursing interventions.

Cullum (1997) identified hundreds of such RCTs, evaluating not only technological aspects of nursing such as critical care, but also other interventions such as patient education. The kinds of questions that need to be asked when appraising an RCT are:

- Was the method by which patients (or clients, nurses, doctors, wards, etc.) were allocated to alternative interventions truly random? Randomisation should ensure that factors other than the intervention which might affect outcome are evenly distributed between the experimental and control groups.
- Was the randomisation concealed? In other words, did the person recruiting for the study know which treatment the next patient would receive? Non-blinding appears to influence the outcome of a study and overestimate the effectiveness of the test treatment (Schultz et al 1995).
- Was the person who followed the patient up and determined the outcome blind to which treatment the patient had received? Knowing which group a patient was in may consciously or unconsciously influence interpretation of how the patient has fared, or even the way in which measurements are taken.
- Was the treatment or intervention under investigation the only difference between the ways in which the groups were treated?
- Were the groups similar at the beginning of the trial, i.e. was randomisation successful in evenly distributing other factors which might have affected outcome across the groups?

The role that critical appraisal skills training plays in the implementation of high quality health care remains unclear. Whilst it might be speculated that teaching health care professionals to track down and appraise research for practice will result in evidence-based health care, there has been little evaluative research to determine if this is the case. A systematic review of the effectiveness of critical appraisal skills training is currently underway at the Centre for Statistics in Medicine, Oxford (see also Chapters 4 and 7).

The Critical Appraisal Skills Programme (CASP) is an Oxford-based UK programme concerned with training health service decision makers and lay people in critical appraisal skills. Half-day workshops introduce participants to the identification and appraisal of research into the effectiveness of health care, and train participants to train others, thus cascading knowledge and skills nationally. By June 1997, CASP had held 216 workshops attended by over 4200 people. They had also trained over 200 people to train others throughout England, Scotland and Wales. The CASP Web page is [http://www.ihs.ox.ac.uk/casp/].

Nurses' and midwives' preferences for dissemination

A number of studies have asked nurses and midwives how they like to read research, and how they would like findings to be presented. One of us (NC) was involved in a study exploring midwives' attitudes to research (Meah et al 1996). The midwives commonly felt that articles in journals were dull and unappealing, used too much scientific jargon, and were not really written for practitioners. Many of the midwives also lacked confidence in their ability to appraise research and make sense of statistics. They preferred the idea of research being disseminated through a combination of a verbal presentation by somebody involved in the project plus a concise report written in plain, jargon-free language. An ethnographic study conducted in Canada reported similar findings: nurses wanted reliable, quick reference material both in print and on computer, and information sources that were available at the site of patient care (Blythe & Royle 1993).

Systematic reviews

Whatever the format in which information is presented to clinicians, it is clear that the information itself must be reliable. Where more than one study has been undertaken in a particular area, there should be a reliable synopsis or summary of the relevant work available. This avoids the need for busy nurses to engage in lengthy and costly literature searching and review (see, however, arguments in Chapter 3 relating to loss of skills). Systematic reviews are reliable summaries of the findings of all the scientific studies in an area; they use a 'systematic approach to minimising biases and random errors' and require that 'the components of the approach (will be) documented in a materials and methods section (Chalmers & Altman 1995). However, the importance of this approach has only recently received widespread recognition. Mulrow (1987), in a review of 50 reviews published in four major medical journals in the USA between 1985 and 1986, used eight explicit criteria to assess their quality:

- Did the reviewer state a specific purpose?
- Were the sources and methods of the search specific?
- Were explicit exclusion and inclusion criteria used?
- Was there a systematic assessment of the validity of the primary research?
- Was the information systematically integrated and the limitations of the data made clear?
- Was there appropriate pooling of quantitative data?
- Was there a summary of the pertinent findings?
- Were specific directions for future research drawn from the review?

It is noteworthy that no review met all eight criteria, only one met six criteria, 32 reviews met four criteria, and 17 reviews met only three criteria. Only one review had clear methods. Mulrow (1987 p 485) concluded that 'current medical reviews do not routinely use scientific methods to identify, assess and synthesise information'. The dangers of an unsystematic approach are that we risk:

- not identifying and recommending care that has been shown to be effective
- recommending care that is ineffective or even harmful.

Common faults with traditional reviews

They only look at published research

The process of publication favours research that is deemed interesting by authors and editors, i.e. generally research that demonstrates statistically significant differences. However, if we only 'see' research which has 'positive' results, we get a biased view.

They are often subjective and uncritical

The findings of any primary research study are only as valid and reliable as the methods through which the research was conducted. Any review must systematically appraise the methodological quality of the primary research under review; it is not sufficient simply to recite the conclusions of previous researchers.

They do not strive to minimise bias

The method by which a review is conducted should be as rigorous as that undertaken for any piece of original research, and every effort should be taken to minimise bias at all stages during the identification, appraisal and analysis of research articles. An important part of this process is the adoption of clear criteria for excluding/including studies at the outset of the review. If resources permit two reviewers should independently review research for its inclusion and exclusion and appraise and extract the data from the articles included. More information on how to conduct and interpret systematic reviews is available in the Cochrane Library and in the guidelines produced by the NHS CRD (NHS Centre for Reviews and Dissemination 1996).

Systematic reviews are most commonly undertaken to explore questions concerning the effectiveness of health care interventions, but may be used to summarise the body of research evidence on any kind of topic. Where several similar studies have measured the same outcome, it is sometimes possible to pool their results in a single estimate of effect. A variety of statistical techniques are available; the overall approach of combining separate studies is termed *meta-analysis*.

Critical appraisal of systematic reviews

It is just as important to appraise the rigour of systematic reviews as it is to appraise original research. A number of different checklists are available to achieve this. For example:

- does the review address a clear and focused question?
- does the methods section clearly describe a comprehensive search strategy which is unlikely to have missed important studies?
- are there clear inclusion/exclusion criteria?
- was the methodological quality of the original research systematically appraised?
- if the individual studies were combined in a meta-analysis, was it appropriate to do so? That is, were the variables to be combined similar across the different studies?

Sources of good-quality reviews

The UK Cochrane Centre and the NHS CRD were established in the 1990s to promote the use of, and facilitate the production of, systematic reviews using a number of strategies. The international Cochrane Collaboration, which is a collection of health care professionals, researchers and consumers of health care who are interested in preparing, maintaining and disseminating systematic reviews of the effects of health care, grew from the UK Cochrane Centre.

The Cochrane Collaboration

The Cochrane Collaboration relies on individuals with interests in particular aspects of health care and a commitment to producing reviews coming forward to participate. There are three main organisational units within the Cochrane Collaboration, viz.

- *Collaborative Review Groups*. Reviewers work with the coordination and support of an editorial team to produce reviews in particular topic areas, for example, stroke, wounds, effective professional practice, schizophrenia, pregnancy and childbirth.
- *Cochrane Centres*. At the time of writing (1998), there are 13 Cochrane centres throughout the world, each playing a particular role. For example, the San Antonio Cochrane Centre in the USA has a special responsibility for the development of the Cochrane Collaboration education and training programme.
- *Cochrane Fields*. There are currently six fields registered: primary health care; health care of older people; complementary medicine; health promotion; physical therapies and rehabilitation; and vaccines. Fields traditionally represent different settings in which health care is

delivered, such as: primary care; groups of health consumers, e.g. older people; or types of health care intervention, such as physical therapies. Although members of fields might undertake reviews, the fields themselves are primarily concerned with identifying trials, promoting the perspective of the field within the work of the Collaboration and disseminating Cochrane reviews to their constituents, for example the primary health care field to members of the primary health care team.

The Cochrane Library

The Cochrane Library is published quarterly on CD-ROM (Update Software, PO Box 696, Oxford OX2 7YX) and contains four databases:

- the Cochrane Database of Systematic Reviews (CDSR)
- the Database of Abstracts of Reviews of Effectiveness (DARE)
- the Cochrane Controlled Trials Register (CCTR)
- the Cochrane Review Methodology Database (CRMD).

The CDSR. This contains the full text of completed Cochrane systematic reviews as well as protocols for planned or ongoing reviews. Many, if not all, Cochrane review groups produce evidence of relevance to nursing, midwifery and health visiting. Examples of completed reviews include:

- adherence with medication
- alternative versus conventional settings for childbirth
- prevention of ankle ligament injuries
- inpatient rehabilitation for hip fracture
- infants' sleep and feeding patterns
- regular aerobic exercise in pregnancy
- training health professionals in smoking cessation.

The CCTR. This is a bibliography of over 100 000 controlled trials which have been identified by contributors to the Cochrane Collaboration. Many of these trials are not listed in MEDLINE.

The CRMD. This database contains over 400 bibliographical references to papers describing the conduct and interpretation of systematic reviews.

The NHS CRD

The NHS CRD has three principle functions:

1. to carry out and commission systematic reviews of research
2. to maintain two databases:
   - DARE
   - the NHS Economic Evaluation Database
3. to disseminate the results of good-quality reviews to the health service.

The DARE. Both before and after the establishment of the Cochrane Collaboration, many excellent systematic reviews on issues of effectiveness had been undertaken by others and published as journal articles and reports. The DARE searches for these high-quality reviews in the international literature and makes them accessible. Each review referenced in the DARE is presented with a structured abstract, and has been appraised for its quality by trained systematic reviewers working at the NHS CRD.

As part of collaborative work between the Centre for Evidence-Based Nursing at the University of York (see Chapter 1 for a description of the Centre) and the NHS CRD, the authors undertook a review of 81 reviews identified through a combination of MEDLINE searching (1987–1994), hand searching of nursing journals (from their inception to 1994), and informal contact with nurse researchers in the UK and abroad. Reviews were obtained for further scrutiny if they appeared to address an aspect of the effectiveness of nursing practice, and/or if MEDLINE or hand searching suggested that they might be systematic. The 81 reviews were divided into those concerned with issues of effectiveness (36), for example 'Effects of preoperative instruction on post-operative outcomes' (Hathaway 1986), and those not concerned with effectiveness, for example 'An analysis of theory–research linkages in published gerontological nursing studies: 1983–1989' (Murphy & Freston 1991). The former 36 reviews were assessed for quality using three criteria. Did the review:

- have a clear question?
- demonstrate a systematic comprehensive search strategy in order to identify as large a proportion as possible of primary studies?
- demonstrate an appropriate synthesis of data?

Nineteen reviews of effectiveness met all three criteria; four reviews met two of the criteria; eight met one criteria; and five failed to meet any of the criteria. Of the 19 reviews which met all the criteria, 12 were published since 1990, suggesting a possible increase in the number and quality of systematic reviews relevant to nursing. All 19 of these high-quality reviews are now indexed on the DARE and the search strategy used by the NHS CRD to identify reviews has been expanded to ensure that as high a percentage as possible of nursing, midwifery and therapy reviews is identified (Droogan & Cullum 1998). The DARE may be accessed through:

- the Cochrane Library
- Telnet to [nhs crd.york.ac.uk]: the user name and password are both crduser
- the World Wide Web at [http://www.york.ac.uk/inst/crd/info.htm]: the user name and password are both crduser
- dialling direct with a modem. Telephone 01904 431732: the user name and password are both crduser.

The NHS Economic Evaluation Database. This contains records of economic evaluations of health care interventions. The structured abstracts detail the methodology, results and conclusions of the studies. This database may be accessed exactly as for the DARE.

The NHS CRD has other dissemination products which include:

- Effective Health Care Bulletins which summarise the results of a systematic review of the clinical and cost effectiveness of a particular health intervention. The reviews are undertaken and commissioned by the NHS CRD (Entwistle et al 1996). The bulletins are aimed at health care decision makers and should be available in NHS and medical libraries in the UK. They are published by FT Healthcare, London.
- Effectiveness Matters which are summaries of systematic or large scale, high-quality RCTs which have been carried out by research teams outside the NHS CRD. Effectiveness Matters are also distributed free of charge within the NHS.
- CRD reports which provide detailed summaries of systematic reviews of research undertaken or commissioned by the NHS CRD. These may be obtained from the publications office, NHS CRD, University of York, York YO1 5DD. Telephone 01904 433634.

Other sources of information. These include:

- The *ACP Journal Club* published by the American College of Physicians, which provides abstracts of high-quality published research relevant to advances in the treatment, prevention, diagnosis, cause, prognosis or economics of the disorders which fall into the category of internal medicine (Entwistle et al 1996). Each abstract is accompanied by a commentary from a clinical expert in the area, who comments on such matters as prior research in the area, quality of the methodology, and possible implications for practice.
- *Evidence-Based Nursing*, which is a quarterly journal produced by the Centre for Evidence-Based Nursing, University of York, UK, School of Nursing, McMaster University, and the Health Information Research Unit, McMaster University, Canada. The journal identifies the best-quality research relevant to nursing that is published internationally, and re-presents these papers as structured abstracts with a commentary on their implications drawn up by a clinical expert.
- *Evidence-Based Medicine*, which is a journal produced collaboratively by the Centre for Evidence-Based Medicine in Oxford and the Health Information Research Unit, McMaster University, Canada. It abstracts good-quality evidence of relevance to general practice, medicine, surgery, obstetrics and gynaecology, paediatrics, psychiatry, anaesthesiology and ophthalmology, as identified from international journals. A clinical commentary is presented with each abstract.
- *Bandolier* (produced by the Research and Development Directorate of

Anglia and Oxford NHS Executive Regional Office in the UK) provides short articles which alert readers to key pieces of evidence about health care effectiveness, and provides a signpost to primary sources. *Bandolier* has a Web page at [http://www.jr2.ox.ac.uk/Bandolier].

Targeting dissemination: the Practice and Service Development Initiative (PSDI)

The *Report of the Task Force on the Strategy for Research in Nursing, Midwifery and Health Visiting* (Department of Health 1993b) recommended that a nursing and midwifery dimension should be incorporated within the review commissioning facility proposed by the NHS Research and Development Programme. As a result the PSDI was established as a part of the NHS CRD in October 1994. It has two objectives:

- to identify and document existing practice and service developments in the UK and to identify key people who are active in promoting these (Droogan & Sanderson 1995)
- to use information collected and the links established with those in practice and service development to help prioritise review and dissemination activity in the NHS CRD.

The PSDI is tackling these objectives through five strategies:

1. a national survey of practice and service developments
2. regional surveys of practice and service developments
3. encouraging networking amongst health care professionals
4. searching the literature for the best available research evidence
5. disseminating the results of high-quality systematic reviews to health care professionals.

The national survey of practice and service developments

A pilot survey was undertaken to provide an initial assessment of the areas of practice and service development. It targeted 1485 health care professionals throughout the UK, 718 of whom returned the questionnaire (response rate of 48%). The top 10 clinical topics where respondents were undertaking developments were: community care; rehabilitation; wound healing; mental health; midwifery; pain; outpatients; clinics; extending professional roles; and cancer. Ninety-nine per cent of respondents stated that they would like to receive research-based information relevant to their area of practice development (Droogan & Sanderson 1995).

Surveying the practice and service developments by region

Following the national survey, it became apparent that regional surveys might offer a more efficient route to identifying the professionals involved and their activities. These regional profiles should provide a more systematic method of data collection and a more comprehensive picture of national developments.

Networking amongst health care practitioners

The information collected in the regional surveys has been compiled into a database of developments. Each NHS library in the regions that have been surveyed has received a free copy of this database, which health care professionals can utilise to contact others working in similar areas. The information collected from the seven regions is held on a database at the NHS CRD, and anyone who would like national information regarding a specific topic may contact the Information Service at the NHS CRD.

Searching the literature for the best available evidence

Searching of the DARE and CDSR is being undertaken by the PSDI to identify systematic reviews which have a message for nurses and allied health care professionals. Reviews with important information for these groups are highlighted through articles which are written for the professional press.

Dissemination activities

Currently, monthly articles are being published in the *Nursing Times* and *Therapy Weekly*, each containing a synopsis of a high-quality systematic review. Effective Health Care Bulletins are disseminated free to members of the PSDI database who are developing practice in a relevant topic area. The NHS CRD and the Centre for Evidence-Based Nursing are currently undertaking eight reviews in wound care and will have completed three by the end of 1998. Wound care is a common topic for practice and service development, and therefore active dissemination of the results of these reviews to health care professionals (in the form of a study day) has been undertaken. During each study day, the best available research evidence in three areas of wound care was disseminated to those health care professionals who have been actively developing practice in these areas. The impact of the study days is being evaluated using pre- and post-tests of knowledge and reported practice. The outcome of this evaluation will inform the development of further dissemination activity.

CONCLUDING REMARKS

Nursing ignores the 'effectiveness' movement at its peril. Whilst nurses must be caring, skilled, empathic communicators, they must also have good evidence for the things that they 'do' to patients. Nurses must be helped to develop strategies for lifelong learning so that they can keep abreast of high-quality research findings without drowning in the literature. Nursing needs more research that evaluates the best way of managing specific situations, and more systematic reviews that summarise bodies of research. However, bodies of research on their own will never be sufficient: we must also develop and test imaginative ways of getting research into practice.

Implementing research and changing practice

'Research is fun, interesting and relevant to practice, yet many nurses do not think of it as any one of these things, let alone all three of them!'

7

Research dissemination and implementation: the role of education

Jill Maben

KEY POINTS

- Research is valued by Project 2000 students and diplomates for the framework and rationale for care it provides
- Poor leadership and lack of support from colleagues in practice demotivates Project 2000 diplomates to implement research and change practice
- Many nurse educators are not research literate and need to be empowered through further research training
- Research should be seen as an integral part of the whole process of both pre- and post-registration education, and not isolated as a discrete entity
- Newly qualified nurses need to be supported and nurtured in practice for their full potential as research-aware practitioners to be realised
- The practice environment should support learning and open discussion amongst staff, with good leadership the key to successful implementation of research in practice

---

INTRODUCTION

Research is fun, interesting and relevant to practice, yet many nurses do not think of it as any one of these things, let alone all three of them! It is clearly a great challenge for nursing education to attempt to change this and create a nursing profession that understands, values and enjoys research so that many more practitioners can see the relevance of it to their own practice. We need intelligent consumers of research (Kramer et al 1981), which means that nurses must acquire the ability to make competent critical evaluations of research studies, thus allowing them to make informed decisions about the care they give (Carter 1996). This chapter will focus upon the role of education in fostering this research awareness, and the dissemination and implementation of research in practice. Pre- and post-registration approaches to enhancing research awareness are examined, and the extent to which these approaches have made a difference in practice form the bulk of the chapter.

BACKGROUND

Currently the gap between theory and practice in nursing remains alive and well. Despite a dramatic increase in research activity and a proliferation of nursing theory over the past 25 years since the Briggs Report (1972), concerns remain that nurses fail to base their practice upon research evidence (Armitage 1990, Bircumshaw 1990, Gould 1986, Lacey 1994, McIntosh 1995). Education is often allied solely with theory, and practice is often deemed to be devoid of theory. Is this true? And if so, why?

The difficulty of translating research findings into practice has been documented by many authors (Carter 1996, Mulhall 1995, Walsh & Ford 1989). Wilson-Thomas (1995) has suggested that it is due to the way in which nursing has evolved that differences between theory, research and education have developed. Research activity is largely concentrated in university departments, and educators and researchers often have little direct responsibility for patient care and so are perceived as remote from practice. This obviously has implications for the utilisation of the research produced (Mulhall 1995). Researchers are seen as idealists, separate from those in the real world, with their own language and jargon which reinforces this view (Ferguson & Jinks 1994, Peters 1992, Reed & Robbins 1991). Other authors have suggested that the culture, history and traditions of nursing militate against the acceptance of research into practice (Close & Cheater 1994, Holland 1993), whilst others have acknowledged that even with the best will in the world, attempting to introduce change can be fraught with difficulties (Close & Cheater 1994, Hunt 1984, McIntosh 1995, Peters 1992). There are clearly several ways to tackle these problems, but the purpose of this chapter is to focus on the role of education in fostering research awareness and the dissemination and implementation of research in practice.

RESEARCH AWARENESS IN THE NURSING CURRICULUM: CURRENT STATE OF PLAY

Education in nursing has undergone sweeping changes in the last decade, one of which has been the introduction of the Project 2000 curriculum (United Kingdom Central Council for Nursing, Midwifery and Health Visiting [UKCC] 1986) which represents a major innovation in pre-registration nurse education. These changes aim to encourage nurses to embrace and build upon a body of knowledge which can inform and improve practice (Orr 1987). Indeed, one of the aims of Project 2000 was to produce nurses capable of reacting to the changing needs of health care into the 21st century. This new type of practitioner should be a 'knowledgeable doer', basing practice on research and providing a sound rationale for the care given (UKCC 1986). In 1988, the government announced the first wave of 13 demonstration sites for the new curriculum and by the summer of 1989, Project 2000 was established. It is now the only way to gain an initial nursing qualification, the final group of 'traditional' RGN students in England having completed their course in 1996. The Project 2000 curriculum was predicted to both enhance the nursing profession's existing qualities and provide the opportunity to use more diverse forms of relevant knowledge (Kendrick & Simpson 1992). Practitioners educated in this way are expected to base their care on research. It was anticipated that these flexible practitioners would challenge others and act as agents of change in practice. The concept of lifelong learning with an emphasis on continuing professional education was also expected to be a product of the new curriculum (Macleod Clark et al 1996).

The Project 2000 pre-registration preparation was conceived as an initial education only, and the emphasis on lifelong learning enshrined in its policy documents (UKCC 1986) helped to facilitate a similar overhaul of post-registration education. The introduction of the Post Registration Education and Practice Project (PREPP) (UKCC 1994) and the Framework proposals by the English National Board for Nursing, Midwifery and Health Visiting (ENB 1990) have been the cornerstone of the changes in post-registration education. Specifically, PREPP requires registered nurses to complete 5 study days every 3 years and to maintain details of their professional development in a personal professional portfolio (UKCC 1994). From April 1992, the ENB introduced a framework for continuing professional education which leads to an ENB Higher Award certificate. This framework comprises 10 key characteristics, one of which is 'the ability to use research, implement and evaluate concepts and strategies leading to improvements in care' (ENB 1990 p 11).

Research training is therefore a component of many post-registration courses with theory based on the latest available data. More specifically, there is an ENB course (870) which facilitates greater research awareness, and graduate studies also fulfil a need in this area (Chapter 4 discusses an evaluation of an ENB 870 course). To specialise further, many nurses are gaining greater research awareness and indeed research training at postgraduate level on master's and PhD programmes which are becoming increasingly popular. However, a mapping exercise undertaken by the Centre for Policy in Nursing Research (CPNR) (1997) indicates that between 1976 and 1993 only 285 doctoral theses relating to nursing were lodged either in the Royal College of Nursing (RCN) Steinberg Catalogue or the Index to Theses held by the British Library. Furthermore, a track record in supervising doctoral work in nursing has been built up in only a small number of centres.

Nursing has been considering the issue of research skills and the implementation of research for a long time. However, it is only more recently, since the medical profession became interested, that these issues have gained greater momentum in the UK. This interest has been catalysed by the evidence-based medicine movement (Sackett 1996) which many, including myself, prefer to call the evidence-based health care movement (see Chapters 1 and 2). It would appear that now the dominant profession (of medicine) is interested, initiatives are developing all over the country and resources are more readily available. The educational packages associated with this movement clearly have relevance for all health care professionals, including nurses. These educational approaches would include teaching critical appraisal skills and the development of journal clubs. The Critical Appraisal Skills Programme (CASP) consists of multidisciplinary workshops. These take the format of an interactive presentation covering what clinical effectiveness is and how it can be researched, the impact of systematic reviews and meta-analysis, and how to appraise reviews in terms of their validity and their applicability to local populations or particular patients. Journal clubs for nurses are beginning to gain ground and often consist of regular meetings of professionals to discuss evidence on which to base their practice. There are little or no data available on how widespread these are, or the form that they take. At least one club known to me in the north-east of England, is run by nurses, for nurses. This club has adopted guidelines from the medical literature (Sackett et al 1997). Work in this club concentrates on all five steps considered fundamental to evidence-based practice (formulate a clear clinical question, search the literature, critically appraise the evidence, implement useful findings and monitor in practice) rather than the aimless repetition of appraising ad hoc papers. Some research course organisers in pre-registration nursing education could learn much from this approach.

Currently there is an unprecedented range of courses related to research, which use a variety of teaching approaches, available to both pre- and post-registration nurses. But is this education making any difference? Do these educational strategies for improving research awareness actually translate into practice? Although this chapter in the main focuses on the Project 2000 course and my own research in this area, before moving on to this I will examine the effectiveness of other educational strategies.

HAS RESEARCH AWARENESS IN THE CURRICULUM MADE ANY DIFFERENCE?

The ability to critically evaluate research studies is vital if nurses are to make informed decisions about research and implement findings within their care. Teaching skills of critical appraisal is the cornerstone of many preferred educational approaches to teaching research awareness skills (McKenna 1995). This has been seen as crucially important in several research studies in the area (see, for example, Armitage 1990, Rodgers 1994). This section will examine the effects of including research awareness in the curriculum, firstly in post-registration courses and then in pre-registration Project 2000 courses.

Evaluating the impact of post-registration courses

In general, the evaluation of post-registration courses and the assessment of methods used in research courses has received little attention (Cavanagh & Coffin 1993). Many researchers recommend various ways of facilitating the uptake of research findings in practice, but few specific courses or educational strategies are evaluated for their effectiveness. In the USA, Harrison et al (1991), in an experimental study of 54 nurses, found that attitudes towards research were improved significantly after an educational intervention which provided research knowledge and skills. The effect was, however, short-lived. In the UK, little evaluation work has been undertaken, but there are some notable exceptions.

The CASP workshops have recently been evaluated (Burls 1997). Pre- and post-workshop questionnaires completed by 3000 individuals from 172 workshops indicated that 86% of participants had gained some knowledge, and for 73% the change in knowledge was considered important. All professional groups (including nurses), except for non-clinical/administrative staff demonstrated a statistically significant improvement in their attitude to research following the workshop. However, the effect of the CASP workshops on critical appraisal skills and decision-making behaviour remains to be addressed (Burls 1997). In addition, a research study day for 19 midwives was evaluated by Hicks (1994). Within the study day, 19 clinical midwives were taught methods of critically evaluating research studies. Two months later, Hicks noted an increase in: the midwives' stated frequency of reading research; their confidence in evaluating research; and the degree of influence that published research had when they reviewed their practice, as well as an increased profile of research for each midwife. Hicks (1994) suggests that it is imperative for the whole nursing workforce to become research-minded, and argues that research skills are essential to all members of the profession.

The Foundation of Nursing Studies (FoNS) organised a series of nine workshops between September 1994 and December 1995, which were attended by a total of 206 nurses, health visitors and midwives. Each workshop ran over 4 days and aimed to teach practitioners the skills and knowledge necessary to critically evaluate research findings and instigate and manage change. Evaluation of the workshops through questionnaires (response rate 84%), telephone interviews and a focus group interview were undertaken. Results indicated that over 90% of participants at seven sites subsequently had the confidence to apply research to practice. The authors conclude that this type of workshop is effective in 'reducing fear and lack of understanding of research, alleviating the problems of jargon and increasing skills of critical appraisal' (Foundation of Nursing Studies 1996 p 11).

The ENB 870 course was evaluated in one university department in 1994–1995 (Lacey 1996). This course, which aims to introduce nurses, mid-wives and health visitors to the research process, has a substantial open learning component (50% of the taught input). Evaluations throughout the course, together with a specially created evaluation 6 months after its completion, were used to assess its impact on the students' practice. The students greatly valued the ability to critically read research and the experience of conducting a small piece of research themselves; these results confirm those from previous studies (Bostrom & Suter 1993, Wright & Dolan 1991). Sixty-five per cent of students had been able to implement research guided by a change proposal developed by each course partici-pant. A growth in confidence related to research and research activity was cited as important by the students of the course. This research is encourag-ing and the author concludes, 'the evaluation...was overwhelmingly posi-tive as regards the effectiveness of the course in influencing practice' (p 300). However, with a 52% response rate for the follow-up questionnaire, the author suggests that questions remain about non-response error (Lacey 1996) (see also Chapter 4).

Post-registration courses build upon the foundations laid in pre-registration education which provide an introduction to research in nurs-ing. Project 2000 aims to produce flexible nurses who are research-aware and maintain a sound rationale for the care they give (UKCC 1986). The next sections draw on data from a project that I was involved with (Macleod Clark et al 1996) and my own recent doctoral work. Both examine Project 2000 students' and diplomates' perceptions of their own research awareness facilitated by the course.

Evaluating the impact of pre-registration Project 2000 courses

From 1992 to 1995, I was involved in a research study commissioned by the ENB which examined perceptions of the philosophy and practice of nurs-ing in the context of Project 2000 in two centres in the north and south of England. My colleagues and I administered questionnaires to students ($n = 498$) at 9-monthly intervals throughout the Project 2000 course in each of the two centres and also interviewed newly qualified Project 2000 diplo-mates in practice ($n = 20$). Much information emerged and the full report contains more details (Macleod Clark et al 1996). This section will concen-trate on the data that related to the students' attitudes to research and the current philosophy of nursing in this respect.

Respondents were asked about general changes in nursing. Over 80% of students felt that nursing in general was changing with the most commonly cited response being related to political National Health Service (NHS) reforms. Over one-quarter of students also cited changes such as greater research awareness and a more knowledgeable practitioner facilitated by Project 2000.

Asked about the significance of nursing research to nursing practice, over 90% of students stressed its importance (see also Chapter 4 for the perceptions of qualified nurses and other health care professionals with regard to research). Research was seen as increasingly important as the course progressed. Reasons for its importance to nursing included the facilitation of quality care, the reduction of rituals, and enhanced professionalism: a move away from the 'this is how we've always done it' approach.

Students valued research for the framework it provided for care. It was seen to provide a rationale for nursing practice and to reduce routinisation. A student, 9 months into the course, suggested: 'Traditional practices can be proved to be of no use and only research can disprove the benefit of certain practices, e.g. rubbing bottoms to prevent bedsores was practised for years and finally proved to be more damaging than not rubbing them'.

Students were subsequently asked about those subjects in the curriculum that they perceived to be of the greatest help in practice, and those which could have been covered in more or less depth. Research increased in importance as a subject of greatest help in the practice area during the course. Only 4% of students at the beginning of the course thought research was helpful, but this rose to 25% 6 months after qualifying. As the course progressed, students were better able to appreciate the relevance of research, and it has been suggested that an early introduction to research provides greater opportunities for socialisation to research in general (Duffy 1986). The early placement of research in pre-registration courses has also been found to increase the use of both research 'content', i.e. results, and research methods in clinical practice (Thiele 1984). However, it is not clear whether those who received an early exposure to research maintained this greater use of research content in their practice than those who had later exposure.

In my study, a sizable proportion of students felt that research was a subject which had been covered in too much depth (8–19% of responses) (Macleod Clark et al 1996). In addition, research was often judged to be badly taught, with little liaison between different lecturers, particularly in centre 2 (south of England), which produced a course that never got beyond defining what research was. Poor teaching does nothing to help nurses view research as being either fun or interesting. A staff nurse who had been qualified for 1 year reflected upon the research teaching component within her Project 2000 course and found it lacking.

I can remember being really disappointed with the research side of it – I can remember thinking on several occasions that the people who taught us research don't know what they're talking about. Unless you know your subject you can't teach it. There was one lecturer – he was brilliant. I snuck into one of his sessions because I was officially in another group, and the difference was enormous.

Despite the difficulties outlined above, over 90% of students thought that research was important to nursing practice. But what happens once the students qualify? Is the research grounding gained on the course enough to help them implement research and change practice as newly qualified nurses?

THE REALITY OF RESEARCH IN PRACTICE: ISSUES AND CHALLENGES FOR PROJECT 2000 DIPLOMATES

This section focuses upon the perceptions and self-report behaviour of the diplomates who completed questionnaires 6 months after finishing the course ($n = 78$) and a subsample who were interviewed at 7 and 11 months after qualifying (Macleod Clark et al 1996). Following on from this study, I decided to examine the reality of practice for the Project 2000 diplomates. Could they implement research, change practice and base their own care upon the theory that they had gained in the course? It seemed a tall order. I sought evidence of Project 2000 diplomates implementing research in practice. I observed and interviewed a number of nurses who had completed a Project 2000 course and who were working in secondary care settings. Four had been qualified 6 months, 1 had been qualified for 1 year and 2 had been qualified for 2 years. Data from this subsequent work are also included in this section.

During the interviews for the first study (Macleod Clark et al 1996), several staff nurses raised the issue of research as a way of both improving nursing practice in general and effecting change in their own practice areas. Knowledge of research was also something that was often expected of them by others, and some 'traditional' nurses were keen to utilise this knowledge. As one diplomate commented:

I think a lot of them expect you to bring all sorts of research-based nursing into practice. In the interviews that I went to as a D grade, everyone said you have had a lot of research in your training, how would you present that research to the ward or how would you change something with research-based evidence? They are much more into that now.

That research could be used to change practice was picked up by a staff nurse at interview, who suggested it to be the way of the future:

I would say that the research-based knowledge is having a hell of a lot of impact on care (. . .) – to raise standards of care, to bring standards in, and to deliver the best care to the patient. I go on all these study days so that I can use the knowledge that I learn from them to bring to the ward setting. So I am actually able to implement change in that respect as well.

From the questionnaire data, the majority of respondents suggested that they were able to relate research findings to their own practice (62% in centre 1 and 72% in centre 2). The most popular areas included pressure area care and pre- and postoperative procedures. The latter specifically included giving information to reduce anxiety and reduce postoperative pain. The perceived benefits of utilising research were the provision of quality care with improved patient outcomes. For those who had been unable to relate research findings to practice (38% in centre 1 and 28% in centre 2), the perceived barriers included lack of opportunity, resistance by colleagues and lack of time.

There was also evidence, from my doctoral exploratory work, of the more experienced diplomates utilising research based knowledge in areas such as pain control, preoperative information giving and wound care. Staff nurse A, who had been qualified for 2 years, suggested:

I couldn't say where I read it, but I've read it that you should use, when the wound's really sloughy and loads of exudate is coming out, you should put it in dry and when the wound's dry, put it in wet, keep it moist – because that's the ideal environment. I mean I've learned that – I've learned what the ideal wound environment is and that obviously comes from research.

Another utilised her own assignments from the course to ensure that her practice in the area of pain relief was based on research. Staff nurse B had been qualified for 1 year:

There's so much evidence to show that good pain relief, that analgesia is under-administered by nurses – certainly when it comes to the use of opiates. So certainly my judgments on when to give Pethidine, when not to give Pethidine, whether you discuss it with the patient, whether you don't, etc. are based upon research

Evidence did not come purely from research (see Chapter 3), and was often either a mixture of research and experience, or was based upon the experience of more expert nurses. Staff nurse A reflected:

Yeah, I think my practice is [research based], but it's mixed a lot in with experience so that the base is research. (. . .) – now I've said 'well research says this works' so I've tried it and then if it's worked then I would have carried on using it, but I'd still be open to other ideas if it didn't work.

The current research base within nursing was felt to be a limitation by staff nurse C who had been qualified for 2 years. She felt that she had almost worshipped research when she first qualified as the only way to do anything. Once she gained more confidence in her own abilities she felt more relaxed:

Now I'm more confident that my knowledge is better and I'm more confident that I know why I'm doing things and that even if things aren't research based they're more practically based, that my biological basis is sounder. So that I don't feel that I have to have such a nursing research base.

Overall I did observe the use of research in practice, and certainly some of the nurses were very committed to the ideas of research and evidence-based practice. The difficulties in implementing research in practice are not new and are well-documented (e.g. Bircumshaw 1990, Hunt 1981) and indeed it would appear that some of the difficulties are the same for the Project 2000 diplomates as they have been for previous generations, for example, limited time to read and study and lack of support and cooperation from other members of the team (Rodgers 1994). The ability to introduce ideas into the practice environment was recognised as an important skill which many diplomates were trying to develop, often in less than ideal conditions. Their ability to act as agents of change, colleagues' resistance to change and the importance of the ward environment are explored below.

Project 2000 diplomates as potential change agents

At interview, many of the qualifiers revealed that they saw themselves as potential change agents. They believed that the course had taught them to question others. Assertiveness and questioning were felt to be assets in trying to bring about change in others, as a staff nurse described:

Towards the end, I started to realise that I did not want to be like some of the nurses out there and I did not just want to cope. I wanted to be able to change things and the only way to change things is by getting other people to change as well. (...) I remember one tutor saying something like, 'You have got to be able to challenge them but you cannot challenge them if you do not have anything to back it up with, so always make sure you know what you are doing.

This was also supported by the questionnaire data. The majority of those who responded (81%) suggested that the course had equipped them with the skills necessary to effect change (see Table 7.1).

Qualified diplomates in centre 2 consistently identified 'research base' more (52%) than those in centre 1 (20%) as one of the skills enabling them to effect change. Having the knowledge to back up action and knowing the rationale behind practice was identified as another principle passed onto the diplomates by the college. Research was often crucial in providing knowledge and rationale for action. One diplomate also emphasised the importance of this for accountability:

Table 7.1 The extent to which the Project 2000 course has equipped nurses with skills to effect change

Category	Centres 1 and 2 (%)
Has not equipped	19
Has equipped	81
Total	100

(n = 78) 6 cases were unable to answer the question

It was always drummed into us from the beginning that you were expected to find out the reasons why you did certain procedures and why you carried them out. (...) If you went ahead and did something and you hadn't a clue why you did it, but just because other people did it, that was no reason to defend yourself.

The diplomates interviewed had both theoretical and research-based knowledge at their fingertips and did not perceive their education to be a 'once and for all' activity. Rather, they were keen to continue learning and to top up their diploma to a degree. By contrast, the newly qualified staff nurses interviewed by Walker (1986) lacked the theoretical grounding on which to base their care decisions. These traditional neophytes had little opportunity for decision making as students and therefore had difficulty as staff nurses deciding upon nursing actions. Indeed, one of the difficulties encountered by them was in deciding when to contact medical staff about a patient's condition (Walker 1986). They were concerned that they often did this for trivial reasons and coped by a process of trial and error, assessing the doctors' reactions. Walker (1986 p 96) concludes: 'the staff nurse appeared not so much to base her decision on her theoretical knowledge of the patient's condition but rather on the reaction of her medical colleagues; a major barrier to any claim for professional autonomy'. The depth and breadth of theoretical knowledge together with the assertiveness training from the Project 2000 course allowed the diplomates to feel comfortable in saying when they did not know how to do something rather than forging ahead on a trial-and-error basis, as had been the practice in the past (Walker 1986). Jowett et al (1994 p 101) reported similar findings from their study: 'the students showed a substantial degree of confidence in their ability to rise to the challenge and were expecting to learn a great deal and to feel comfortable about asking in the workplace. As one of them elaborated: 'I think Project 2000 people may be less afraid of saying that they don't know something'. This I have conceptualised as 'no bluffing' (Maben & Macleod Clark 1996a) – an aspect of the patient-centred approach to care where diplomates would not jeopardise patient care or safety, and took accountability very seriously.

Decisions concerning patient care were an issue for the diplomates in this study, but tended to revolve more around a lack of experience than an absence of theoretical knowledge. This may be common to any neophyte or indeed anyone commencing a new job. Indeed, the staff nurses displayed an understanding of theory and research which often surpassed that of their more experienced colleagues. As students, they had been attempting to base their practice on theory and research since first stepping into practice, often finding themselves at odds with colleagues and being forced to justify their actions. The implications of this are threefold. Firstly, this influenced the confidence levels of the diplomates. Secondly, it directly affected their relationships with their colleagues, and lastly it ensured that the patient/client was at the centre of care delivery rather than at the mercy of routinised practice. Areas of difficulty did exist, however, one of the most prominent of which was colleagues' resistance to change. This may have been particularly marked in our study (Macleod Clark et al 1996) since we focused on a group of early diplomates from one of the original demonstration districts, and data were collected in 1993–1994. The issue of resistance may have lessened over time in these original sites, but remains where Project 2000 students and diplomates are a more recent addition to the workforce.

Structural difficulties in implementing research: colleagues' resistance to change

Project 2000 diplomates are educated to question and challenge practice, and to utilise research. As Jowett et al (1994 p 105) note, 'the extent to which they were critical of routine practices for which no other rationale other than tradition could be found was striking'. This is in direct contrast to Lathlean's finding that the newly qualified staff in her study tended to 'accept established clinical procedures uncritically and to demonstrate a very limited knowledge of research' (Lathlean 1987 p 26). In the study by MacLeod Clark et al (1996), some of the diplomates' nursing colleagues offered some resistance to these new ideas, causing conflict, and at times difficulties and stress, for the new staff nurses. Perceived differences between themselves and their 'traditionally' trained colleagues were explored as a possible reason for some of these difficulties.

Newly qualified nurses were asked: 'As a qualified nurse to what extent, if at all, do you see yourself as different from non-Project 2000 trained nurses?' A smaller percentage in centre 1 as compared with centre 2 saw themselves as different from nurses who were not trained through Project 2000 (see Table 7.2).

Respondents' open comments, added after they had completed the Likert-type responses as shown in Table 7.2, continued to back up this variation in response between the two centres. However, as shown in Table 7.3, the most frequently cited type of difference perceived by the Project 2000 respondents was the same for both centres: a category labelled 'thirst for

Table 7.2 The percentage of diplomates who perceive themselves as different from 'traditionally' trained nurses

Category	Centre 1 (%)	Centre 2 (%)	Both (%)
Not different	60	48	56
Different	40	52	44
Total	100	100	100

Table 7.3   Perceived differences between Project 2000 and 'traditionally' trained nurses

Category	Centre 1 (%)	Centre 2 (%)	Both (%)
Thirst for change	31	50	37
The same	29	21	27
More training/academic input	24	46	31
Less practical experience	22	25	23
Different approach to patient care	20	4	15
Broader knowledge base	10	8	9
Other	18	8	15

For both centres 1 and 2 there were 75 respondents and 117 responses, as each respondent could write more than one response

change'. This encompassed notions of both research awareness and a questioning approach with rationale for actions.

Almost half of the cohort did not, however, perceive great differences between themselves and their colleagues who trained before the advent of Project 2000. It was suggested that whilst the knowledge base may be different, with respect to research, Project 2000 and traditionally trained nurses were integrating. Some diplomates found that traditionally trained nurses were using them as a resource for research knowledge, but PREPP was reducing any differences in knowledge.

Offering opinions and challenging the ideas of established staff was perceived at first by the diplomates as difficult, although they found it somewhat easier to challenge peers. The wards appeared to operate on hierarchical levels, where a D grade junior staff nurse was not in a position to challenge sisters or consultants. This is in keeping with the warning offered by Ryan who proposed that as a strategy for change Project 2000 was giving 'the greatest responsibility to the weakest and most inexperienced group'. (Ryan 1989 p 15). There may be a tension for the Project 2000 diplomates between holding onto the beliefs and values gained from the course, often appearing 'different' from colleagues, or compromising their view of nursing in an attempt to fit in and be accepted in the workplace (occupational socialisation). It has been suggested that Project 2000 has been constructed 'back to front': 'the students have been given the function of educating the clinical areas; rather than the clinical areas being enabled to prepare students for a new model of practice' (Ryan 1989 p 1). Ryan contends that it endows learners with everything they need to fit in with present practice, except the capacity to change it.

One staff nurse who I interviewed was investigating the literature concerning different pressure-relieving mattresses, as she felt that the one currently used in her practice area was an infection risk. She was under no illusions, however, about the difficulties she might face in bringing about any change:

Table 7.4   Ability to influence practice in area of work

Category	Centre 1 (%)	Centre 2 (%)	Both (%)
Able to influence practice	48	56	51
Unable to influence practice	52	44	49
Total	100	100	100

Again, it is not something that I could broach or I do not feel I could broach it with the sister at the moment, because that is her theatre, her water mattress. (...) she will not give a thought as to why she is doing something. It is just that it is done like this and that is that. I give the surgeons what they want, they are happy with it and that is that. That is fine but there are other bits that she should really take on board but you do not mince words with sister.

The questionnaire data provide further insight into this. A mixed response was obtained to the question 'To what extent have you been able to influence practice in the area in which you work?' (Table 7.4). (Chapter 4 includes a discussion of how far other groups of qualified staff have been effective in influencing practice.)

For those who suggested that they were not able to influence practice, being too junior or inexperienced was the most frequently cited response (26% in centre 1 and 32% in centre 2). In centre 1, staff were perceived as more open and receptive, and the qualifiers there were more willing to challenge others and share ideas. In both centres, however, when asked how they would like to change practice in their work areas, the most frequently cited responses were:

- to increase research-based practice (26% in centre 1 and 33% in centre 2)
- to change old attitudes and practices (21% in centre 1 and 19% in centre 2)
- to have more individualised care (15% in centre 1 and 15% in centre 2).

As outlined above, there was some evidence of research being utilised in practice. However, as my doctoral exploratory work proceeded it became clear that examining research-based practice for this group of nurses, and indeed for those in their first year of registration, was part of my agenda and not theirs. For them it was important to get to grips with their new role and learn the range of skills they felt they needed to be staff nurses. These included dealing with relatives, planning their own and others' work, discharge planning and familiarisation with medication and its administration. Their needs lay in these other areas which centred around support and preceptorship, and this has been demonstrated by other work (Maben & Macleod Clark 1996b). The need for support and the impact of the ward environment on their ability to practice as they had been taught is explored in the following section.

Structural difficulties in implementing research: support and the ward environment

The first few months after qualification was an extremely traumatic time for the new diplomates as they felt the weight of responsibility and accountability that their new uniforms bestowed (Maben & Macleod Clark 1996a). Many felt very unsupported and thrown in at the deep end. Staff nurse D had been qualified for 6 months and found her first experience as a qualified member of staff so traumatic that she had left to seek employment elsewhere in a more supportive environment. She reflected upon her initial experience:

I think you need to have a supportive place for your first post. That's the key, because from feeling good as a management student I lost all my confidence in my first few weeks and I was just a gibbering wreck in tears all the time and that just wasn't me and it wasn't fair to make me feel like that.

The newly qualified nurses that I spoke to felt physically and emotionally drained and found little time for reading or keeping updated. Research in this situation was either tucked away to be used at a later date when they were on their feet or was put off until they were no longer 'just a D grade' and had more authority in the face of often unyielding colleagues. As the staff nurses progressed in their careers, however, research-based practice again often took a low priority as they became too demotivated in poor environments to change practice. Staff nurse D illustrates the importance of a supportive environment. Having left her initial post (described above), she sought an environment which reflected her own philosophy of nursing and where she felt able to challenge peers and suggest that practice be based on what she knew to be good theoretical evidence. She described undertaking a leg ulcer dressing with her preceptor:

my preceptor started doing the bandaging, and he was bandaging from the knee down to the ankle, and I'm thinking, 'Do I say something or not?' And I thought 'I'll go for it,' so I said 'Actually, I think you're supposed to put pressure from the ankle towards the heart so you're promoting the venous return'. I knew that for a venous ulcer you needed to promote the circulation and that to bandage from the knee downwards would be completely pointless and there would have been no point in doing the dressing in the first place to do that.

In this more open learning environment, her preceptor was able to learn from her, a newly qualified nurse, and she felt more able to express her opinions than she had on her first ward where she had felt very unsupported.

Keeping motivated

For those who had been qualified longer than 6 months, maintaining the motivation to continue to implement research into practice revolved around the individual nurse and the presence of facilitating factors in the ward environment. For these diplomates it included supportive, well-motivated colleagues who were prepared to listen and try new ideas, together with good leadership. Staff nurse A compared her own ward area where she described attempting to implement change as 'banging your head against a brick wall' to the environment in which her flatmate worked:

everyone around her is very motivated, they're all using a research-base – bringing research into the working environment and they all want to give. They haven't got stuck in ruts – they aim to give the best possible care and they'll look at everything to do that. They won't just carry on with what has been fine for the last 10 or 20 years. So she's drowning in books at home and she's really, really motivated to keep going.

She went on to contrast their reading materials at home:

She had all these books and she says I'm going to do some reading – and I get out a *Marie Claire*. (...) I am envious of her working environment because they push them all to do things, push them on courses. Whereas here you fight to get on anything and the ward is so pushed to do everything.

Staff nurse C, who had been qualified for 2 years, suggested that she had tried to implement an infection control policy for central lines but that poor ward management and lack of communication between staff meant that this often broke down. This significantly demotivated her towards attempting to change practice in her ward area:

When I first qualified, I felt that I tried to take too much of the research issues on myself and I felt very responsible for my own practice (...) that I should be absolutely research based about everything. Whereas now I feel that there's no point in me being research based about something if the rest of the ward isn't working in the same way because at the end of the day it doesn't do the patient any good. It's my responsibility to ensure my own practice, but it's not my responsibility to set up research things for the entire unit.

In summary, the diplomates I interviewed and observed appeared neither to 'fumble along' (Walker 1986), having a theoretical and research-based framework for their care, nor to 'get through the work' (Melia 1987) at all costs. They seemed more able to hold on to the nursing values as taught in college by putting the patients first at all times. The move away from an apprentice-orientated training towards a more professional model based in a higher education institution may have facilitated a different socialisation process which may help explain these differences. Research is definitely more on the agenda of diplomates of the Project 2000 course than it was on mine as a newly qualified staff nurse in the early 1980s. The Project 2000 diplomates – who now form sizable chunk of the nursing workforce and will be increasingly so – have an understanding and knowledge of research which is unsurpassed in the history of nursing in the UK. With a greater focus on supporting practice development, their enthusiasm and knowledge in this area could be put to better use. Preceptorship and support for these diplomates is crucial if their initial enthusiasm is to be harnessed for the good of patient care. It is useful to unpick this research knowledge and identify some of the key skills needed for research awareness and the dissemination and implementation of research in practice.

KEY RESEARCH SKILLS AND ATTITUDES

Students and diplomates of the Project 2000 course appear to possess a number of key skills and attitudes which may help facilitate the greater integration of research and practice. These encompass both broad-based and specific research skills which may be helpful to others wishing to improve their own practice.

Broad-based skills and attitudes

- assertiveness skills
- a questioning approach to practice
- a desire to have a rationale for all nursing actions
- a basic understanding of the research process and its language coupled with an ability to search for and interpret research reports/findings
- a desire to continually learn – not to see the pre-registration course as a 'once and for all' education – and a willingness to admit to a lack of knowledge.

Specific research skills and attitudes

- ability to formulate clear clinical questions
- ability to access and retrieve literature manually and from databases
- ability to search the literature
- knowledge of research language and terminology
- critical appraisal skills
- basic knowledge of quantitative and qualitative research methods
- ability to synthesise knowledge, often from disparate fields
- ability to implement useful findings
- ability to reflect on practice and monitor research in practice.

KEEPING THE MOMENTUM GOING

The role of education in promoting research-based practice is complex and varied. This chapter has focused primarily on pre-registration education and in particular the role of the Project 2000 curriculum in fostering research awareness. It would appear that research is on nurses' agenda to a far greater degree than it has been in the past. The Project 2000 curriculum moves nursing towards an all-graduate profession, and the framework,

PREPP and higher award changes to post-registration education have all played a part in this. The greater academic focus within nursing has also undoubtedly helped with a desire to have a credible research-based profession, and more recently the 'evidence-based medicine' movement has pushed evidence-based decision making to the forefront of health care.

This section will now turn to three key issues which appear to be central to many of the issues that confront the Project 2000 students and diplomates in relation to research-based practice. Aspects of these key issues also have relevance for other educational interventions and for nursing in general. They include:

- the preparation and role of nurse teachers
- the need to nurture newly qualified nurses
- the development of practice areas.

Preparation and role of nurse teachers

The move towards evidence-based care and the changes implicit in the Project 2000 and PREPP reforms present challenges on many fronts to nurse teachers. Most evident is their ability and willingness to engage in providing the education required to create research-aware and research-active practitioners. The Strategy for Nursing Research in England (Department of Health 1993b) suggests that the status and quality of research in nursing will rest largely on the quality of academic advice and supervision. The report recognises that 'the number of academic staff in colleges and university departments of nursing, health visiting and midwifery is currently limited and must be expanded' (Department of Health 1993b p 14). This implies a need for both further education of staff and a raising of the research profile of nursing (Cavanagh & Tross 1996).

Nurse teachers are clearly a key group in increasing research knowledge within the nursing profession, yet attention to this important part of their role is often lacking. Clifford (1993) undertook a small questionnaire survey with nurse teachers ($n = 40$, response rate of 60.6%) which revealed that over 50% of respondents felt that they did not have adequate preparation for undertaking research work. Indeed some respondents felt that research was poorly understood by members of teaching staff who were involved in supervising learners! This lends support to a survey undertaken in Northern Ireland in which 43% of a sample group of 70 nurse tutors had received no research training and 26% had only attended individual study days (Murray et al 1990). Similarly, Walker (1993) found that many nurse educators were not research literate. Clifford & Gough (1990) suggest that these findings are not surprising given that most nurse educators are themselves products of traditional nurse education where research studies were not even addressed. Clifford (1993 p 52) further suggests that 'the situation should give cause for concern to a profession that is placing its trust in nurse teachers to ensure that sound knowledge base in research is developed in students under the guidance of nurse teachers'.

Research undertaken by the ENB (Le Var & Steadman 1996) found that by 1994, 70% (n = 6163) of nurse and health visitor teachers had achieved degree status, with an additional 22% reading for a first degree. In midwifery the figures were 48% (n = 657) and 32% respectively. In the same year, 22% of nurse and health visitor teachers had obtained higher degrees with a further 22% studying at postgraduate level, whilst the corresponding percentages for midwifery teachers was 14% and 27% respectively. However, Kirk et al (1996) suggest that the possession of a first degree alone is not sufficient to confer academic credibility in the higher education context where the vast majority of staff will have a higher degree. They also question the necessity for all teachers to acquire research skills apart from those necessary to critically appraise research reports. Current moves within nurse education, however, would suggest that this would need to be the majority of nurse teachers. Logue (1996) expresses concern over this and argues that the role of the 'teacher' is being eroded by nurse teachers being pressurised to undertake research when many of them neither wish to, nor are competent to do so. He also confirms Clifford's (1993) findings by suggesting that there is an 'increasing trend in nurse education for teachers with little or no skills, knowledge or experience in research to be expected not only to undertake research but to teach it at pre- and post-registration levels' (Logue 1996 p 67). Nolan (1989) suggests that there is a two-tier theory–practice gap. On the first tier is the gap between what educators know and teach and up-to-date research findings, and on the second tier is the gap between what educators know and teach and what students and others practice.

There is also a lack of clarity about the best ways to teach research (Cavanagh & Coffin 1993, Clark & Sleep 1991, Kramer et al 1981, Overfield & Duffy 1984). There are many factors that may influence student's attitudes to research (Eckerling et al 1988) and there is an urgent need for research into the different teaching approaches used in developing research skills. One of the most obvious issues is for nurse teachers to make research interesting and compelling to students so that they are not turned off it, i.e. make it fun! There is evidence that some teachers treat research as a separate entity and compartmentalise it (Hunt 1987, Macleod Clark et al 1996). The integration of research into the curriculum would appear to be a reasonable goal. Research should be seen as an integral part of the education process in all pre- and post-registration nursing curricula, not isolated as a separate entity (Closs & Cheater 1994). Work undertaken before the integration of colleges of nursing into higher education has suggested that an absence of a research culture and the failure of research to guide nurse teaching are two of the reasons why research fails to influence clinical practice (Clark & Sleep 1991, Hunt 1987, Smith 1979). With recent changes in the structure of nurse education, this may no longer be the case. However, many of the teachers in the newly amalgamated colleges of higher education will be the same individuals. Logue (1996) offers four categories of teachers in relation to research, those who:

- can do research and do
- cannot do research and do not
- can do research and do not
- cannot do research and do.

It is the latter categories which give most cause for concern. If nurse teachers are to continue teaching research, there is a need to clarify the preparation and support they require in this role (Clifford 1993). Nurse teachers have a key role to play in the dissemination of results and in producing students who are critical consumers of research (McKenna 1995). Failure to address the quality of research teaching and the development or empowerment of teachers to undertake the role will result in a continuing gulf between the rhetoric and reality of research-based practice (Clifford 1993).

Nurturing the diplomates: preceptorship support and supervision

The research work that I have been involved in over the last 5 years has convinced me of the need for adequate support and supervision for all nursing staff, but especially for the newly qualified diplomates. These nurses emerge from their Project 2000 courses full of hope, enthusiasm and optimism about their careers as nurses, only to feel frustrated, disenchanted and unsupported only a few weeks later in many cases. It would appear to be important that nurses are initially nurtured if their full potential is to be acknowledged. In a recent review of the literature, it has been suggested that the support of colleagues and superiors is the most important determinant of behavioural changes in nursing practice (Francke et al 1995). Indeed, the authors draw upon several studies (e.g. Brasler 1993, Suitor Scheller 1993) to suggest that a continuing education programme may have little or no effect if colleagues in the practice setting show disapproval or are unsupportive. I would argue that the situation is exactly the same for those emerging from the Project 2000 programmes.

It has long been realised that a programme of support may facilitate the transition process (Kramer 1974, Lathlean et al 1986, Maben & Macleod Clark 1996a, b, Shand 1987). This has also been recognised by the UKCC (1993) who have suggested that support and guidance should be available for a period of approximately 4 months to all newly qualified staff nurses in the form of preceptorship. It would appear from my work (Maben &

Macleod Clark 1996a, b) and other studies (Jowett 1995) that this has not been realised.

For diplomates to feel comfortable about challenging peers, be able to utilise their research-based knowledge in practice, and indeed to learn from the experience of others, they need first to be nurtured into the complex role of the qualified nurse. Some authors have suggested that a preceptorship programme does not aid the qualified nurses' socialisation process (Itano et al 1987) or produce any significant difference in the clinical skills of preceptored and non-preceptored nurses (Huber 1981, Myrick 1988). Morton-Cooper & Palmer (1993), however, suggest that the aims and outcomes of any evaluation of preceptorship must be clearly stated at the outset. Is preceptorship seen primarily as a means of helping individuals adapt and conform to their work roles; as a mechanism for supervising and enhancing work performance; or as a support role intended to ease the transition to clinical work with a view to reducing stress and 'reality shock'? They suggest that some evaluations of preceptorship have been unclear as to the specific aspect of preceptorship that was being evaluated. It is important to state that the role of preceptorship in North America is primarily to enhance role performance, whilst the support aspect of the role is at present considered to be of importance in the UKCC's proposals (1993). In the UK, preceptorship is taken to be 'a form of educational relationship which is intended to provide newly qualified (or returning) professionals with three things: access to an experienced and competent role model; a means by which to build a supportive one to one teaching and learning relationship; and a smooth transition from learner to accountable practitioner' (Morton-Cooper & Palmer 1993 p 99). These authors have argued effectively in their work that preceptorship is both fundamental to the transition process and long overdue in the UK. They suggest that the strengths of preceptorship lie in 'enabling practitioners to develop their knowledge and skills in an atmosphere of trust, with colleagues who have experienced it for themselves, and who have been prepared for and understand the challenges confronting the beginning practitioner' (Morton-Cooper & Palmer 1993 p 100). Preceptorship therefore allows new nurses to grow into their role, feel supported, and develop the use of research in practice.

Diplomates who have received preceptorship have found it extremely valuable, and all the newly qualified diplomates who I interviewed felt that it would have been helpful, even if they had not experienced it (Maben & Macleod Clark 1996b). Allen (1993) has also suggested that a period of preceptorship is valuable. Having experienced a particularly supportive preceptorship herself, with consistent and clear boundaries, she suggests that this has enabled her to 'push the boundaries of community nursing and to think radically about what it is that district nurses do' (Allen 1993 p 60). Robinson et al (1993 p 34) suggest that new staff nurses need 'a period of time in practice to consolidate what they have learned and gain confidence with the support and guidance of a skilled and experienced mentor'. They go on to recommend a development programme whereby for the first 3 months at least, a new staff nurse should not be left in charge, and during which time skilled mentorship should be available. It is perhaps lamentable that the UKCC has not made preceptorship mandatory, but more importantly, what is required is a recognition and commitment from the profession that preceptorship is both desirable and necessary. For, as Jowett points out, 'creating a structure without securing staff commitment was not of benefit to the recipients' (1995 p 6). Indeed Robinson et al (1993) recommend the need for further education and support for the preceptors of the newly qualified diplomates themselves. This would seem crucial, particularly with respect to their knowledge and experience of research. The role of lecturer–practitioner is emerging as a means of resolving the problem of appropriate clinical supervision, and where the development of the role is clearly understood, it has been highly successful (Vaughan 1989).

If support and preceptorship are not forthcoming in the early days and weeks after qualification, it is easy for the new diplomates to become extremely stressed and anxious. Many of those who I interviewed described thoughts of leaving nursing at this stage, or having to treat it as 'just a job'. In these instances, implementing research in practice becomes a low priority in a situation where getting through each day and surviving is paramount. The support received or not received in the transition period is crucial to the future of nursing, as the first 6–12 months may set the staff nurses' pattern of future practice. If they are not well supported and well received, they may either abandon the questioning approach gained on the course and 'fit in' or choose to leave nursing altogether. Kramer's seminal work (1974) on nurses' socialisation identifies this as 'withdrawal', that is, finding themselves unable to maintain their college values in the work-place, they seek an alternative practice environment where they hope to be able to practice as they had been taught, or indeed they leave the profession altogether. Either of these options would appear to be undesirable for the nursing profession. A national survey of 4321 (72%) registered nurses with RCN membership appears to support this. More than one-third (36%) of NHS nurses said that they would leave nursing if they could. The ability of the NHS to recruit newly qualified nurses has diminished over the 1990s. Only 89.7% of the 1995 registration cohort were in nursing in their year of registration and 86.2% of them in 1996. This compares to 98.6% in 1991 and 95.2% in 1992 (Seccombe & Smith 1997). Furthermore, the proportion working outside the NHS in the second year after registration continues to rise. These are worrying trends, and ways of reducing wastage from the NHS should be examined. This is a complex issue, beyond the scope of this chapter, but the research that I have been involved with would suggest that preceptorship, support and indeed supervision for all staff would be of value. Clearly, however, other factors impinge upon the ability of nurses to implement research in practice. Some suggestions for narrowing the theory–practice divide are examined next.

Bridging the theory–practice divide: development of education and practice areas

The theory–practice divide has been shown to militate against the implementation of research-based practice in many ways. There are various means of tackling these issues and many are beyond the remit of this chapter. I would like, however, to briefly draw upon some of the literature to examine some suggestions for bridging the gap from both an educational and a practice perspective.

Education

Ferguson & Jinks (1994) have argued for a full-scale and multidimensional overhaul of the curriculum. This would involve creating a multidimensional model which involves a joint planning approach by education and service staff with the aim of facilitating integration of what is taught with what is practised. Jordan (1994) suggests that one of the challenges for education is to develop programmes which assume that all individuals, not just an elite, can become competent thinkers. The recommendation of the Committee on Nursing (Briggs 1972) remains relevant today, and in order to achieve the recommendations put forward, post-basic education must expand to encourage a dialogue between theory and practice (Jordan 1994). She further suggests reflection in action (Schon 1987) as a strategy for encouraging this dialogue, in which the concrete experience of the nurse becomes the 'learning peg' on which to hang abstract concepts/theory.

Closs & Cheater (1994 p 765) suggest that research has become included in the pre-registration curricula (Project 2000) to a greater or lesser degree, yet 'little attention appears to have been given to the area of research utilisation'. In 1993, Bassett called for commitment and effort from nurse education and practice leaders to work together to find ways of creating more realistic opportunities for practical experience in research utilisation. This could be facilitated through mutual respect of each others' strengths and skills. Castledine (1994) similarly advocated a clinical appointment based in both practice and education, that is, an expert clinical lecturer who could liaise between practitioners and educationalists. It has also been argued that researchers need to be seen to have clinical credibility if their findings are to be regarded as relevant to practice (Castledine 1994). In 1994 the UKCC expressed their commitment to nurse teachers remaining more closely in touch with nursing practice through the PREPP proposals. Others have suggested that this would enable teachers to give more practice-based tutorials (Castledine 1994, Dale 1994). Lecturer–practitioner posts which seek to combine the roles of clinician, lecturer and researcher have been operating for many years in some education establishments and trusts (e.g. the Oxford Radcliffe Hospital NHS Trust). They are now becoming more widespread and may help redress the balance and bridge the theory–practice gap. However, currently there is a paucity of evidence indicating the effectiveness of these posts.

Practice

Practice development is also crucial if research is to become more widely available and utilised. The depth and breadth of literature in this area is beyond the scope of this section, and only that pertinent to the Project 2000 case is considered here. For further examples in the literature see, for example, Closs & Cheater (1994), the Conduct and Utilisation of Research in Nursing (CURN) Project (1983), Funk et al (1989), and Wilson-Barnett et al (1990). Chapter 9 also provides examples of the reality of practice-based development in the clinical setting.

As outlined earlier, Ryan (1989) has argued that Project 2000 in many ways has been constructed 'back to front'. He suggests that 'the students have been given the function of educating the clinical areas; rather than the clinical areas being enabled to prepare students for a new model of practice' (p 1). For the full potential of the Project 2000 diplomates to be realised, it is necessary to think about creating an environment ready to receive them and ready to utilise their skills to the full. Ryan (1989) has proposed a 'support hierarchy' model rather than the current command hierarchy as best accommodating the needs of Project 2000 students and diplomates, and being more beneficial to patients. The support hierarchy model facilitates a patient-centred approach to care. He suggests that with the patient at the apex, the relationship between all the primary carers, e.g. family, nurse, doctor, is a collegial one, with each supporting the others. This is appealing as a model of organisation, but requires some fundamental changes in the whole health care system for it to function effectively. Others, however, argue that it is the role of education to lead practice and to set goals; 'ideals' may therefore be useful and 'important for transmission of knowledge to the learners and students of the discipline' (Norris 1982 p 35).

Diplomates have suggested that a supportive environment includes not only preceptorship, but forward-thinking, dynamic staff (Macleod Clark et al 1996). This was felt to be an especially important quality in the ward sister/manager whose position of authority ensured the ability to change practice and implement new ideas. The importance of the role of the ward sister in facilitating a learning environment has long been recognised (Fretwell 1982, Orton 1981, Pembrey 1982). Together with more senior managers, ward sisters have a responsibility to the new diplomates in attempting to facilitate an easier transition process. The diplomates also stressed the importance of staff respecting and trusting them, and giving them appropriate responsibility. A forum for discussion and regular feedback from colleagues was also seen as a vital part of a generally supportive environment (Macleod Clark et al 1996).

Describing the clinical support available to Project 2000 students in the form of mentorship, Wilson-Barnett et al (1995) suggest that an understanding of this complex issue requires examination of the broader clinical environment. Students identified staff committed to teaching, a good team spirit and practitioners with time to give to students as factors facilitating good learning. Teachers in the study added that being encouraged to ask questions, a lack of hierarchy in the team, and staff with a positive view of Project 2000 were also important (Wilson-Barnett et al 1995). Phillips and colleagues (1993) support this. They investigated the assessment of competencies in nursing and midwifery education and training. The research process was found to be instrumental to the process of learning, with the best means of developing and refining professional judgment, including assessments of competence, being through research and education. 'Nurses and midwives who are both "knowledgeable doers" and "reflective practitioners" are found most often where research-based professional practice is institution wide and all members of the community are engaged in a process of action, reflection, critique and further action' (Phillips et al 1993 p 3).

CONCLUSION

This chapter has outlined the role of education in facilitating a move towards research-based practice, and has drawn on work in the area of pre-registration education. Clearly there have been some moves forward with a greater research awareness, and in some instances this has translated into nursing practice. Much of this has been facilitated through educational developments, not least the development of a greater academic base for nursing through Project 2000 and the move into higher education. There remain a number of challenges ahead, however, not least a change in nursing culture and indeed in public perceptions of nursing. Have we gone far enough yet? Should we be moving towards an all-graduate profession or will changes best be wrought in the practice environments? Nursing and the wider society have yet to reconcile themselves to their current relationship with academia as evidenced through the continual attacks on the credibility of Project 2000-educated nurses in the press (Lawson 1996, Rayner 1997). Knowing how to utilise academically prepared nurses remains a challenge for those within and outwith the profession. This warrants serious attention, which as a profession we should address before it is too late.

ACKNOWLEDGEMENTS

The author is indebted to the students and qualified nurses who took part in the studies. The study of Macleod Clark et al (1996) was commissioned by the English National Board for Nursing, Midwifery and Health Visiting and the doctoral work was undertaken through support provided by the Smith & Nephew Foundation. The views expressed are the authors' and are not necessarily those of the English National Board or of the Smith & Nephew Foundation.

8

Creating change in practice

Anne Mulhall

INTRODUCTION

The first seven chapters of this book examined some of the major issues concerning the dissemination and use of research in nursing, and attention to these will be vital if progress is to be made in closing the research–practice gap. However, practitioners can develop a positive attitude to research, they can acquire the skills to critique studies, and they can be provided with a supportive environment, but nothing will actually happen unless someone, somewhere, initiates change. The final phase of the research to practice model described in Chapter 1 is implementation, and implementation of research will require changes to practice. These changes may act in a very individual way and be almost imperceptible. Thus practitioners who have been enthused with the idea of research at a workshop may begin to view their work in a different light, become more questioning of practices that they have taken for granted, or begin to look at 'problems' from a number of different, or new, standpoints such as feminist theory. Other changes may be much more tangible and involve many people, both managers and direct care givers, in drawing up new strategies and guidelines for the way in which nursing care is provided. Some examples of these sorts of changes are provided in Chapter 9. It is evident, however, that this stage of closing the research–practice gap is problematic. We may motivate ourselves to acquire new skills, we may adapt our attitudes, but ensuring that those things make a difference to the ways in which we practice, and what is more the ways in which our colleagues practice, is more difficult. Actions and sustainable actions are always much harder than words!

In Chapters 2 and 4 we saw that although practitioners from a wide range of specialities viewed research positively, fewer of them actively used research to change practice. Some of the reasons why the implementation cycle fails to come full circle to bridge the research–practice gap were also discussed. Central to many of the difficulties that the research–practice gap presents is the issue of creating and managing change. For if new evidence is to be implemented, then very often practice must change. If nursing care was provided by a bank of programmable machines, then the only question related to change that would arise would be: who is doing the programming? Fortunately, care is not provided in this way, but unfortunately (for change managers at least), the involvement of people in care provision ensures that making changes is a complex and often frustratingly difficult exercise. Why should this be so? To start to answer this question we must first look to what happens when we try and change things.

WHAT HAPPENS WHEN CHANGE IS PROPOSED?

The word 'change' can of course be used as a noun or a verb. In the former sense it usually alludes to something that has happened: an outcome. For example, a change in care delivery from team to primary nursing would indicate that a different way of delivering care had been instituted: primary nursing had been substituted for team nursing. In a way, once a change has become established it ceases to become a change and becomes part of accepted practice or procedure. As a verb, change relates to a process: something may be changed to, from or into something else. Whilst established changes may cause difficulties, it is usually the process of change that creates the greatest challenge, and whatever else it does or does not do, there is no doubt that change challenges. It challenges individuals, organisations and social structures, and it is usually the process of change which causes the greatest challenge.

Change challenges

Although each of us possesses our own set of attitudes and beliefs, we are placed within the wider system of shared ideas, concepts, rules and meanings of the particular society in which we exist. This culture tells us both how to view the world and how to act in it. Cultural forces are exceptionally powerful and lead to what sociologists would term 'normalised behaviour'. In other words, unless there is some compelling reason not to, human beings tend to think and behave in ways consonant with the prevailing cultural norms. Change may challenge those norms and call into question beliefs and attitudes which currently 'glue' the social system together. Not surprisingly this intervention is usually viewed as a threat to the integrity of the system and the individuals within it. Jill Maben's research into Project 2000 diplomates discussed in Chapter 7 illustrates clearly how changes in the system for nurse education may be viewed as threatening by nurses who were trained earlier, on more 'traditional' courses.

In *Nursing Rituals: Research and Rational Actions*, Walsh & Ford (1989) argue that much nursing practice lacks a rational basis and ignores research findings. Although empirical work would support their claim that nurses often fail to use research to underpin practice (see Chapter 2), it is hard to see why they consider this to be irrational. For, in a subsequent book (Ford & Walsh 1994), they suggest a number of plausible reasons to explain this situation, including problems with nurse training, gender stereotyping, the immature state of research, stress defence mechanisms, and the influence of attitudes and beliefs. Bearing in mind the comments above about cultural forces, from this perspective, so-called ritualistic nursing practice and the reasons why nurses are reluctant to abandon it could be viewed as perfectly logical.

In a wider sense, rituals serve a protective and stabilising function: they tell us about the values of our society and how it is organised. Rituals occur in many settings and in many forms, they are not just about religious cere-monies. Health care work is replete with rituals: the consultant's grand round; the nursing handover; the first antenatal visit. Such events take place at defined times and in certain places, where everyone 'knows' what the codes of behaviour, dress, matters to be discussed, etc. are. If change is introduced then the normal order of things may also change. For example, Savage (1995), in her ethnographic work on two hospital wards, explains how consultants were reluctant to support primary nursing because they no longer had a focal point (the charge nurse) through which to organise their work. They resisted the change because the system with which they were both familiar and content altered. Not every piece of research that is implemented in practice occasions such major organisational changes, but with every change, someone somewhere, be it the staff nurse, the porter, the supply manager or the ward clerk, will have to make some minor or major adjustments to the way in which he or she goes about his or her work.

Who is affected by change?

The simple answer to this is everyone, but not just as individuals. Particular groups of individuals, for example student nurses, may be affect-ed, as may be the 'fabric' of the particular society. Thus change challenges not only individuals, but the wider organisation and the social structures that uphold it. At the interface of care delivery, a proposed change in prac-tice may both threaten individual practitioners and make them feel guilty – hasn't my practice up until now been satisfactory? Could I have done more for my clients if only I had read that research paper? Change may also cause increases in workload or changes to the pattern of work. For exam-ple, an innovative one-to-one midwifery service radically altered the work-ing patterns of community midwives (Cresswell 1997). Furthermore, individual patients and clients may be highly resistant to proposed changes: that wound bandaging, urinary catheter, anti-embolism stocking, works for them; why should they change it on the evidence of a research study undertaken with other people?

Individuals may also react to change as part of a group. This is most obviously illustrated in the conflicts that arise between the professions of nursing and medicine. Walby et al (1994) studied this by interviewing 262 nurses and doctors in five hospitals about: the boundaries between their areas of responsibility; their perceptions of interprofessional teamwork; and issues that had recently caused conflict. Almost half of the recorded incidents of conflict related to questions about professional boundaries. In particular, there were certain areas of care, such as wound management and control of elimination, which nurses perceived as firmly within their professional boundaries. Yet although a nurse may decide what to put on a wound, in certain cases a doctor will be needed to agree to the prescription. It is not difficult to see that nurses trying to implement research-based change in this area may run into problems if their medical colleagues disagree with their proposed treatment strategy, and there is much anecdotal evidence to confirm that this is so. Furthermore, this reaction to a potential change is not merely about differences in professional opinion over particular treatments. Very often, determining where these professional boundaries lie and defending them helps to constitute what is distinctive about the different professions, and so the reaction to the proposed change is also symbolic.

From an organisational standpoint, the implementation of research may cause changes to the way in which services must be arranged, the sort of equipment that is needed, and the type of staff skill mix required; even the physical layout of the hospital, clinic or health centre may need to change. Thus although research-based change may save money, there may also be considerable resource implications. In addition, the implementation of research may create a different environment or ethos in an organisation. This may be seen as very beneficial by some staff and patients, but for others it may (1) not be consistent with their beliefs and attitudes and (2) cause them to change their working practices. For example, Dorothy Baker (1983) in her research describes how the sister of an elderly care ward (Sister Green) decided to 'allow' patients to make their own decisions regarding when they wanted to get up, wash, have breakfast and so on. This changed the ethos of the ward by flattening out the power hierarchy between the staff and the patients, since the latter now had more control over their daily lives. However, the new system only actually operated when Sister Green was on duty: the night staff and the doctors were unhappy with the new way of working and eventually Sister Green left and the system returned to its original state.

Change may also affect the social structure of health care delivery settings such as hospital wards, health centres or nursing homes. The example shown earlier in the Chapter illustrates how the introduction of primary nursing changed the relationships and standing of various 'actors' in the health care scenario, both staff and patients. This disrupted the usual pattern of culture and caused a number of difficulties as people attempted to come to terms with the new order of things. Change may thus alter the power relations both between and within professions, and with the clients who are receiving nursing care. This may challenge individuals' authority to make decisions, alter their areas of responsibility and generally under-mine their former professional standing.

Systems theory proposes that the elements in a system are interrelated and interdependent: a change may have effects well beyond the original area in which it was introduced. Implementing research will create changes to the way we organise and deliver nursing care, but as we have seen, these changes may act in both overt and more subtle ways, and ripple out to affect not only other individuals, but groups of individuals and the very structure of the health care environment in which we work.

CAN CHANGE BE MANAGED?

If change is such a complex process which can have serious ramifications beyond its original point of input, it seems reasonable that attempts should be made to manage it in a rational and logical way. Certainly a significant volume of work has accrued in the organisational management literature concerning change management. The first part of this section will explore how this literature has perceived change and has suggested strategies for its management. However, it is perhaps testament to the following quota-tion which is attributed to Machiavelli, the 16th-century Florentine philoso-pher, that despite this ever-burgeoning literature, the introduction of change is still so consistently mismanaged:

There is nothing more difficult to take in hand, more perilous to conduct, or more uncertain in its success than to take the lead in the introduction of a new order of things.

The organisational development approach to change

La Monica (1994) defines change as the moving of the system from where it is (the actual) to where we want it to be (the optimal). This definition of change neatly encapsulates the approach that many of those working in the organisational development tradition have taken (see, for example, Beckhard & Harris 1987, Plant 1987). Briefly, this approach suggests that managers (and it usually is general managers) firstly identify where their organisation should be and whether change is necessary, through an analy-sis of the current demands for change (these could be from consumers, the government, etc.) and through recourse to the mission statement defining the organisation's raison d'être. An assessment is then made of the present state of the organisation, which is contrasted with the desired future state (as in La Monica's definition above). How to move towards this new state is then explored by determining the sorts of changes that will be required, the readiness and capacity of the organisation to change, and potential bar-riers which will prevent the change. An activity plan may then be devised.

During the implementation phase of the plan, it may be necessary to facilitate the changes through perhaps the provision of appropriate training and the active management of resistance.

This model of change management is referred to as linear since it assumes that the process of change proceeds through a simple step-by-step approach from one stage to the next. The thinking behind it stems from positivistic science, and also the assumption that the social world and the people in it are rational and logical. The organisational development approach has strongly influenced management theory in the UK, and the introduction of general management into the National Health Service (NHS) has resulted in this type of model being increasingly applied in health care settings (Spurgeon & Barwell 1991). Furthermore, nursing management may follow the lead provided by general management. Wilson (1992) illustrates how the nursing management of a large Canadian hospital was strongly based upon a positivistic and mechanistic world view.

The foundation for the organisational development movement was laid by Kurt Lewin (1951) through his well-known force field theory of change. This proposes that change is the product of forces which are either driving or resisting a change. Figure 8.1 provides an example of how his theory may be used to look at the forces which are either driving or resisting a move towards more evidence-based practice. It is derived from suggestions

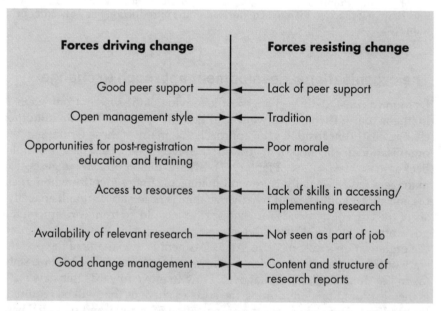

Figure 8.1   Lewin's force field theory of change, illustrating the forces involved in increasing evidence-based practice in nursing.

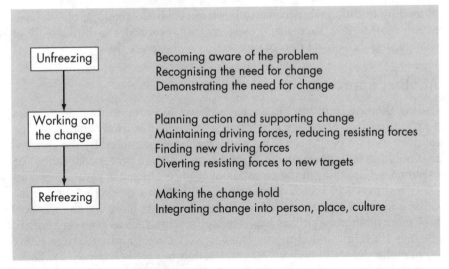

Figure 8.2   Lewin's three-phase model for change.

put forward by a group of nurses who were attending a research utilisation workshop. Lewin also suggested a three-phase model for achieving change through manipulating the equilibrium of the force field model (Fig. 8. 2). Firstly, the current state must be 'unfrozen' by becoming aware of the problem and the need for change. Secondly, the change must be worked on by increasing the forces that are driving the change and minimising the forces that are resisting the change. Finally, the situation must be 'refrozen' with the change integrated into the person, the organisation and the culture. However, a number of approaches to planned change are now found under the organisational development umbrella (see Spurgeon & Barwell 1991 for a review).

In a more radical departure, Pettigrew (1985) has attempted to expand the analysis of change as an isolated event to include a focus on historical, cultural and political factors. Studying organisational change at ICI, Pettigrew's research emphasises how change should not be viewed as a prescribed intervention, but as the culmination of external pressures combining with internal management action. Change occurs when a subset of people in the organisation become aware that the present state of operation is not compatible with what is happening in the wider world. To achieve the change it then becomes necessary for these people to delegitimise their opponents' ideas through a subtle building of support within the political and cultural systems of the organisation. Change then occurs as an outcome of power struggles between different interested parties, rather than as a result of strategic planning and managerial goal setting.

Despite their differences, these two approaches to change are underpinned by traditional business studies theory which largely adopts a positivistic world-view. There are, however, other approaches to thinking about change, and the second part of this section will explore these.

Another approach

During the last 15 years, nurses have begun to examine various theories and approaches to research which go beyond the traditional scientific model based on positivism. This move has been prompted by the concern that nursing, both as an academic discipline and as a profession, cannot be explored solely through the methods of science, since it encompasses concepts and practices which do not fit neatly within a predictive, universal, cause and effect type model. Thus nurse researchers have begun to undertake more qualitative studies based on approaches such as phenomenology (Benner 1984), grounded theory (Melia 1982), ethnography (Savage 1995), ethnomethodology (Lawler 1991) and action research (Hunt 1987). These approaches are concerned with trying to explicate the meaning of certain phenomena which are studied 'in their natural state', hence they are referred to as being in the interpretist/naturalistic paradigm. Box 8.1 outlines the differences between these two approaches. In contrast to the natural science paradigm, many, but not all, qualitative designs are built around the supposition that it is not possible to control the bias that a researcher brings to a study. Rather, such bias must be recognised and articulated. Partly due to this idea, and also as a result of their 'liberationist' underpinning, much qualitative research is also concerned with the positioning of the researcher versus the 'researched'. But what has this got to do with change theory?

Box 8.1   Paradigms or world-views which may inform health care research

Positivists consider that the social world, just like the physical world, is orderly and rational. Thus, although people think, have feelings and communicate, this is not perceived as a barrier to the scientific method. It is thus possible to determine universal laws which help us to predict and explain phenomena. Positivists propose the idea of an objective reality independent of the researcher and they strive to reduce any bias that might occur when collecting data. Data are usually quantitative.

The other major paradigm is *interpretitism/naturalism* which is concerned with understanding human meanings and studying phenomena in a 'natural' state or 'as they are'. It takes a different view from positivism by suggesting that a measurable and objective reality separate from the researcher does not exist. Therefore the researcher cannot be separated from the 'researched'. Who we are, what we are, and where we are will affect the sorts of question we pose, and the way we collect and interpret data. These 'biases' must be acknowledged and explored during the research process. Furthermore, from this world-view, social life is not thought to be orderly and rational; knowledge of the world is relative and will change with time and place. Research approaches here try to capture the whole picture, rather than a small part of it. Data are usually qualitative.

The relevance of nursings' expansion of its research paradigm to our discussion of change lies in some of the ideas that underpin these other ways of viewing the world, for nursing has extended these ideas beyond research to develop some alternative ways to conceptualise change and to think of different ways to introduce change within practice. Three areas are worthy of further discussion here, namely:

- critical theory
- feminism
- action research.

Critical theory and feminism

Critical theory emanated in the 1920s from the Frankfurt School of Sociology which was influenced by Marx's critique of capitalism and the class system as the restraining forces in society. However, in later years, culture rather than economics was conceptualised as the constraint (Habermas 1970). A central assumption of critical theory is that society is structured by meanings, rules and habits which are adhered to by social beings (Allen et al 1986). The purpose of the theory is to unmask those aspects of society that restrict or limit human freedom and maintain the status quo. Before 'critique', the social world is presented and accepted as a natural phenomenon. Critical theorists propose that reflection on the rules and traditions that uphold the way we think and go about nursing work will facilitate an examination of taken-for-granted assumptions. But how will this help with our attempts to introduce change? Critical theory will be helpful on two broad fronts. Firstly, subordinated cultures (as nursing is) tend to take on the characteristics of the dominant group. Simply possessing a knowledge of critical theory will alert nurses to this fact, and to the influence that it may exert on their realisation of the need for change. Secondly, in practising critical reflection, nursing will be able to expose the social structures that maintain things as they are, and thus come to a more insightful analysis of how change might be effected.

Like critical theory, feminism is also committed to emancipatory goals, but here the focus is on gender. In a female-dominated profession which has organised its philosophy and activities around a traditionally feminine attribute – caring – it is not hard to see that a concern with gender is crucial. Speaking of nurse education, Thompson (1987 p 35), asserts that '... it usually provides a strong liberal worldview consistent with white middleclass male ways of defining reality'. Raising the collective nursing consciousness to such issues is critical to any reasoned strategy for change. Feminist researchers are also much concerned about the relative position of researchers and 'researched'. They are conscious of the unequal partnership that exists between themselves and their informants, and constantly reflect on this (Skeggs 1994).

Both feminism and critical theory, then, express concern about subordinated groups and suggest mechanisms by which their voice might be heard. In terms of change theory, these ideas provide a very different perspective from the organisational management theories outlined in the section above. This is classically conceptualised as the difference between the bottom up approach, as epitomised by feminism and critical theory, and the top-down approach advocated by the positivist thinking which lies behind much managerial theory.

Action research

Action research is defined by Carr & Kemmis (1986 p 162) as '... a form of self reflective enquiry undertaken by participants in social situations in order to improve the rationality and justice of their own practices...'. Classically described by Lewin (1946) as a problem-solving approach framed around a spiral of steps which include planning, action and evaluation, action research has evolved to include a number of models: the technical collaborative; the mutual collaborative; and the enhancement approach (Holter & Swartz-Barcott 1993). Meyer (1995) outlines this evolution of action research from the functionalist perspective of Lewin through an interpretative phase into a new paradigm perspective which emphasises practitioners as researchers, self-reflection and the development of critical thinking (see above). Echoing the principles of feminist research and critical theory, the new paradigm research perspective is concerned with 'doing research *with* and *for* people rather than *on* people' (Meyer & Batehup 1997 p 175).

From this description of action research, it is not too difficult to see how such an approach would be useful in managing change. Indeed, one of the main aims of action research is to create change and improve practice. For despite their differences in philosophical underpinning, Newton (1995) suggests that all the models include the main characteristics of action research, namely: collaboration between researcher and practitioner; identification and resolution of problems; changes in behaviour; and theory construction.

In summarising this section, it is perhaps useful to return to our opening question: can change be managed? The above discussion has explored this by contrasting the theoretical positions taken by the top-down and bottom-up approaches to change management. However, although each approach is embedded in a fundamentally different world-view, and each advocates quite a different model of achieving change, both are actually premised on the assumption that change is possible. Moreover, although in theory these two positions can be clearly distinguished, in the messy world of practice it is less clear how firmly these theoretical models are enacted. The last section of the chapter will attempt to ground these ideas more closely with the reality of everyday practice and grapple with some of the dilemmas and pragmatics that bedevil our attempts to effect change.

OPTIMISING CHANGE: WHAT WORKS

Every book on management in health care includes a chapter on change, and many texts have been devoted entirely to this topic. Yet despite this, probably every health care worker in the country could cite examples of changes that have been badly managed. Indeed, one of the constraints to research-based practice emerging from our study of nurses' and managers' attitudes to research (Le May et al 1998) (see Fig. 2.1 and Box 2.2 for details of this research) is the continual barrage of change within the NHS that health care workers are having to accommodate. Pattison (1996 p 257) provides a salutary list of change mismanagement principles which stem from his experience as a chief officer of a community health council negotiating with a regional health authority. Examples include 'Be surprised and hurt when other groups and people attack or question your intentions... This helps to create a communication barrier and may prevent awkward questions...' and 'Do not explain immediately, openly, and clearly what you want to do and why... In particular do not admit that the changes proposed have anything to do with resource distribution or cuts'. Sadly, such examples are not just tongue-in-cheek, but represent the experience of the author and probably many others. As Pattison (1996 p 258) remarks 'It is not enough for enthusiastic managers to adopt simple schemata for managing change and then expect other people obediently to pursue the leaders' vision of a better future'. There are, however, no easy answers. It is clear that changes, both large and small, are an integral part of 20th-century life. What we need is a more realistic and sensitive notion of what change is, how it manifests itself, who is affected, and how we can optimise its challenge to everyone's benefit. This final part of the chapter will start to address these issues by an exploration of some of the problems of trying to change practice in the NHS. These will be set against some tentative proposals for a more useful change management strategy.

Problems of change in the NHS

This chapter has already hinted at some of the potential problems associated with change in general. Those arguments will be expanded here, with specific attention given to change in the NHS. The discussion will cover the following topics:

- conceptual problems with change
- issues of power
- barriers to research-based practice.

Conceptual problems with change

As mentioned previously, the rational, linear model of change has been frequently evoked in the NHS and it has to be said it holds an intrinsic appeal. However, this almost certainly relates to its perceived simplicity as a logical series of steps, or recipe for successful change. As Spurgeon & Barwell (1991) note, this approach is unrealistic in its expectations since real life rarely proceeds in an ordered fashion, and decision making for planning is not well prescribed. Furthermore, Ford & Walsh (1994) point to the inflexibility of such models and their dependence on each link of the chain holding for success. Other commentators (Braybrooke & Lindblom 1963) argue that the entire approach is flawed, since, in their opinion, complex decisions cannot be made by rational and systematic evaluations of alternative strategies for change. Rather they should proceed through making small incremental improvements on the current situation. This elicits a scenario where managers do, and should 'muddle through'. Such notions are congruent with sociological ideas that change is frequently unintended and occurs outwith the control of individual actors within any social situation.

It has also been suggested that since people do not act rationally and logically all of the time, the linear rational model is unfeasible (Sheehan 1990). However, this stance makes certain assumptions about rationality, and the position of those who define what is and what is not rational. Rationality is relative; in other words, we are all rational in our own worlds. You may know that the research evidence suggests that a new wound dressing is more effective than the one your client is using, but if the client is happy with the current product, it is reasonably effective, and a change is likely to cause him or her distress, then you will make a rational decision to continue with the old product.

Another set of problems about change relates to whether theories and models developed for the private sector have any currency in public sector organisations like the NHS. Gunn (1989) argues that the latter have multiple goals which must be attained within specifically demarcated areas of activity and against a backdrop of values which are fundamentally different to those of the commercial world. Managers in the NHS must juggle the needs of central and local government alongside the general public interest for an equitable, consistent and accessible service. Those factors which may legitimately drive change in the private sector may not therefore be present in the NHS, even with the advent of the internal market. As Pattison (1996 p 255) comments, 'When it comes to a large non-profit making organisation with a long, socially appreciated tradition of providing services to all citizens it could be said that radical change is contraindicated'.

Finally, conceptualisations of change in the NHS must be viewed in the light of prevalent Western ways of viewing the world. The current ethos emphasises the importance of the individual, of moving forward, developing, changing. Management texts are redolent with enthusiastic strategies for planning and leading for a better future. Thus change, far from being a morally neutral category, takes a mantle of progress, and progress towards a greater good. In this type of culture, resistance to change becomes morally unacceptable. Those who create barriers to change are perceived as holding up the natural order of things.

Issues of power

The French philosopher Michel Foucault argued that, within the construction of social order, power and knowledge are interdependent. The power to know comes with words and discourse, which in their turn constitute power. For example, medicine has become a way of thinking which has considerable influence and much authority throughout society. How did this happen? Foucault (1976) discusses how, in reducing the body to a medical entity subject to physical examination within the confines of a hospital or clinic, diseases could be identified and named. This knowledge of disease and pathology brought with it power and legitimisation by the state, such that medicine now holds a highly influential position in the social order. Although, as we shall see later the powerful position of medicine is germane to some of the arguments related to changing practice in nursing, it is the principle of power/knowledge that is important here.

Within the NHS, certain groups of professionals hold more power than others. Historically, medicine, through a strategy of occupational closure, state support and the creation of a unique body of knowledge, has consolidated its power base. However, the reorganisation of the NHS and the demise of consensus management (whereby doctors, nurses and administrators participated in collaborative planning [see the Salmon Report 1968]) may now be contributing to a decline in the dominance of medicine. Driven by a political concern with cost containment, general managers have now become a powerful force within the NHS. Whilst some would consider that nursing has been successful in its struggle for professional status (Abel Smith 1960), others suggest that medical control is still highly evident (Witz 1992). As with medicine, the implementation of the Griffiths Report (NHS Management Enquiry 1983) significantly eroded the power base of nursing by removing nurses from key management teams. Nursing is thus subordinated to both medicine and general management.

This discussion of power and how it is constituted is important to considerations of change, for the power structure of the NHS determines 'whose voices, purposes and aims are privileged, who determines the nature of change, and who will benefit from it' (Pattison 1996 p 255). The idea that competing groups of individuals have more influence on the course of change than any planned management strategy was demonstrated by Pettigrew's influential research at ICI discussed earlier in this chapter. The arguments presented here indicate that, much as the profession would wish it to be otherwise, it is clear that the introduction of change in nursing practice will be significantly influenced by other groups. This will almost certainly lead to a conflict of interests and resistance to the proposed change. It might be argued that this would only be the case in certain circumstances where, for example, nurses and their clients were being disadvantaged, and that the subject of this book – research implementation – would be free of such connotations. However, the nature of evidence for practice, its 'level', and who decides what is and what is not legitimate knowledge is highly contested (Chapter 3 discusses these issues at greater length). This indicates that a recognition of power issues is extremely important in optimising change related to research, and this will be expanded on later.

Barriers to research-based practice

Much of what has been said already in this chapter either has been based on the theoretical literature or has drawn on examples of research from disciplines other than nursing. To balance this and to ground the discussion more closely in practitioners' experiences, I would like to outline some of the barriers to research-based practice which emerged from a qualitative study of nurses' and managers' attitudes to research (Le May et al 1998). The design of this study and some of the other results are discussed more fully in Chapter 2. Boxes 8.2 and 8.3 summarise the issues that practitioners and managers respectively perceived as restraining their efforts to make research-based changes to practice.

The barriers to change covered a number of themes ranging from individual attitudes and beliefs to educational issues and professional relationships. Similar themes have been reported by others (Rodgers 1994). However, a new finding was the fact that although individuals admitted deficiencies in their own research skills or a fear of research, 'negative' attitudes were often attributed to others. Previous studies have identified members of other professions, such as doctors as managers, as blocking nursing efforts (Funk et al 1991, Lacey 1994, Rodgers 1994), but several of our respondents suggested that it was their nursing colleagues who created barriers to instigating research-based practice: either 'older' nurses who were unwilling to change practices that had served them well for many years, or colleagues who made disparaging remarks concerning respondents' attempts at continuing education (see also Chapter 7).

Managers' perceptions concerning research utilisation have received little attention in the literature. For managers in our study, the nature and history of the organisation were very influential. Thus, mental health and community trusts were perceived as 'Cinderella' disciplines which may not attract dynamic researchers who might create evaluative cultures that

---

Box 8.2 Barriers to research-based practice as perceived by practitioners

Attitudes
- Lack of cooperation
- Lack of motivation
- Fear
- Resistance to change/ritualised practice

Typical quote
'There is fear and apprehension, mistrust, just another fad idea for the nurses on the ground.'

Beliefs
- Research will not make a difference
- Research data are not appropriate
- Conviction that current practice is OK

Typical quote
'If we started total research-based practice would we do things differently? I don't think we would.'

Professional relationships
- Medical staff block implementation
- Medical staff consider nursing research substandard
- Nursing colleagues are uncooperative
- Senior staff are resistant to change
- Research should be undertaken by practitioners
- Research 'goes' with an individual
- Low grading of research staff

Typical quote
'Simply because it was not carried on through. I felt they played a game of research really.'

Organisational issues
- Time
- Pressure of workload
- Too much change

Typical quote
'The nurses on the ground feel that it might be another imposition on them from above, because of all the changes that are going on in the NHS at the moment. I think that is why nurses are suspicious of anything. . .'

Educational issues
- Practitioners unaware of or unable to access research
- Lack of skills in critical appraisal
- Research reports are jargonistic

Typical quote
'It is not couched in terms that are manageable, and I think they get tired of new catch phrases, and it is the different way things are spruced up.'

---

would foster research-based change. Managers also recognised the effect of health service reorganisations and their constant culture of change, which was seen as detrimental and destabilising. The problem of the internal market stifling the sharing of evidence-based practice was also mentioned. There was also some controversy concerning continuing education and its failure to link to trust objectives. This nicely illustrates some of the points raised above concerning power, for it is likely that managers were con-

---

Box 8.3 Barriers to research-based practice as perceived by managers

History/nature of the organisation
- Not being a teaching hospital
- Research not part of culture
- Community and mental health trusts have special problems

Typical quote
'We are not a big teaching hospital obviously and we do not have a big research infrastructure involved.'

Reorganisation of the NHS
- Directorate structure
- New initiatives/too much change
- Competitive marketplace
- Drive for efficiency: time for reflection or meetings lost

Typical quote
'. . . something that would change practice, then I think it would be very wrong if people were keeping that to themselves. But nevertheless the sort of market situation has meant that there are a lot more things that people keep what you might call commercially sensitive.'

People issues
- Research is 'attached' to individuals; no trust strategy in place
- Critical mass of research-minded staff needed
- Medical dominance

Typical quote
'One of the difficulties is that you have to have the right people there. . .with looking to people to lead things, if that person goes you lose momentum.'

Staff development and education
- Cost and rationale of changing education
- Academic training is not related to trust objectives
- Training is not evaluated
- Academic input is not sustainable under normal work conditions

Typical quote
'The benefit to the individual is that they have developed these research skills, but what was the ultimate spin off for the trust?'

---

cerned that the research agenda should more closely align with corporate goals and focus on topics related to efficiency and effectiveness: the priorities of general management, but not necessarily of nursing.

Making change happen

At the beginning of the chapter, it was noted that if research was to be implemented then very often this would require change. The changes might be wide-ranging and affect many individuals within an organisation, such as the example of the introduction of primary nursing, or changes might be on a more personal basis, and even at a cognitive rather than a behavioural level. This chapter has examined a wide-ranging literature concerning change and situated it within the province of nursing. Three essential requisites to optimising change in general, and research-based change in particular, emerge. Effective and sustainable change to nursing practice can only occur through:

- a framework that incorporates a more sophisticated awareness of how the social structure of the NHS affects change
- a clearer statement of the evidence that nursing needs for effective practice
- a strategy and context that provide nurses and nursing with adequate resources to effect change.

Most research in the area of implementation indicates that nurses are aware of the need to base their practice on the best available evidence (see also Chapters 2 and 4). That many of them do not do this is tied up in an intricate web of individual, political and socio-cultural barriers which conspire either to prevent change even being initiated, or to stymie it once started. The remainder of this chapter will expand on the three themes above to explore how change might be handled more effectively within nursing.

A more sophisticated awareness

At a practical level, nurses who are eager to make changes in practice based on sound research will be extremely frustrated if their nursing and health care colleagues and/or the organisational set-up of the workplace prevents their achievement of this goal. Jill Maben, in her chapter on research and education (Chapter 7), vividly illustrates some of the difficulties that newly qualified diplomates encountered in their attempts to ensure that practice was research based. However, it is my argument here that for change to proceed, individual practitioners must become more sophisticated in their analysis of what the effects of their action may mean. They need to take on board some of the theoretical arguments rehearsed above which relate to the possession of power and what makes certain groups more powerful than others. Whether we like it or not, nursing is in a subordinate position: what we need to do is acknowledge this and critically examine what it means to our efforts to effect change. This leads us to another theoretical idea, but one which may provide some cheer! It is the concept of standpoint epistemology (epistemology being the theory of knowledge, or how we come to know what we know) (see also Chapter 3).

According to Nielsen (1990 p 10), standpoint epistemology 'begins with the idea that less powerful members of society have the potential for a more complete view of social reality than others, precisely because of their disadvantaged position'. That is, as a sort of survival strategy, subordinated groups must be attuned to the ideas of the dominant society in which they exist, but alongside this they also hold an awareness of their own group's views (a so-called double vision). The classic example of this is of course the case of women in patriarchal societies, but the model might equally well be applied to nursing's position viz-a-viz medicine/management in the health service. One only has to think of the ways in which nurses often have to organise their care around the preferences of particular surgeons and yet still attempt to integrate their own conceptualisations of good care, to see how this idea might apply. The concept of standpoint epistemology would suggest, therefore, that nursing has the potential to be more knowledgeable than, say, medicine or general management concerning the social realities of attempting to create change. We will return to this subject at the end of the chapter.

A second idea that needs articulating here concerns the concept of autonomy, for it seems that in thinking about making change happen, individual, and indeed group autonomy will be very important. Walby et al (1994), in their study of the working relationships between doctors and nurses (see earlier in this chapter), record some highly relevant information about the ways in which the two different groups conceptualise the idea of a 'professional'. For doctors, a professional is someone who takes responsibility for his or her own actions, who acts as an individual and who makes his or her own judgments. Rules, procedures and regulations are thus seen as restrictive. This view of the autonomous individual is in contrast with nurses' accounts, which emphasise that a professional is accountable for his or her practice but is guided to this end by rules and surveillance by senior professionals. Therefore, although both professions speak of autonomy and professional accountability, it is clear from Walby et al's work that these concepts may mean different things to different people (see also Chapter 3). In working towards change, this is another aspect that we need to take into account: the notion that the historical legacy and current working practices of the different professions may profoundly affect the ways in which ostensibly universal concepts, such as autonomy, are conceived and thought about. Resistance to change can be drastically reduced if a genuine attempt is made to see the situation through other people's eyes. However, the evidence from empirical work such as that cited above is often needed before such considerations become obvious.

Being sure of the evidence that nursing needs

Currently there is tremendous pressure on both the profession and individual practitioners to base their practice on rigorous evidence. However, in Chapter 2 I started to raise the idea that there are certain problems about what constitutes rigorous evidence and who defines what this category might include. Thus in exploring the sort of culture of research that might be developed in nursing, we come up against difficulties in accommodating some of the 'untidy' things such as emotions and feelings within the traditional natural and social science paradigms. An understanding of the physical body is essential, but this must be complemented by evidence from the social sciences because, as Lawler (1997 p 48) so perceptively notes, '…we also practise with living, breathing, speaking humans'. Furthermore, knowledge for practice also comes from both our professional and life world experiences. Thus nursing, through its particular relationship with patients and their sick or well bodies, will rely on different sorts of evidence and different ways of knowing. These ideas are also discussed in Chapter 3.

With regard to the project for change, it is crucial that we begin to articulate these arguments in a cogent way beyond the nursing arena. It has to be made clear why nursing needs to draw on this eclectic body of knowledge and these different ways of viewing the world. The penalty for not doing this and falling under the yoke of an entirely biomedically driven evidence-based agenda, will be an even greater reluctance on the part of nurses, health visitors and midwives to change their practice as a result of research. If research is not even framed within the types of world-view that make sense to practising nurses, then there is little hope that they will find it of relevance. A commitment to changing practice will only be achieved through a much deeper engagement with these ideas, and an ideological shift by those who are currently driving the movement for clinical effectiveness. Even from a practical standpoint, it appears from the outside that particular strategies, which if further developed might surely have the potential for enhancing research-based change such as action research, are given short shrift in the current world of research funding (Meyer & Batehup 1997). This is despite the value of action research being highlighted in a key document exploring consumer issues in the NHS (Blaxter 1995).

The two requirements for change outlined above concentrate very much on issues of social change, of ways in which nursing might become more sophisticated in the way it both recognises the restraining forces and presents its needs to others who occupy more influential positions. In a way, this echoes recently raised arguments that nursing's allegiance to the concept of individualised care has led to the subversion of the more perspicacious insights that sociology might bring (Cooke 1993), and the counter-argument that there is no reason why nurses must reproduce this ideological consensus (Porter & Ryan 1996). Instead, as the latter authors illustrate, nurses have the option of adopting a critical stance (see earlier in this chapter for an explanation of critical theory). However, on a more practical note it is clear that changes in practice will seldom occur without the support of adequate resources. Indeed Porter & Ryan's case study concludes that the theory–practice gap on the ward that they studied was largely the result of insufficient resources restricting nursing theory being effectively implemented in practice.

Resources for change

Porter & Ryan (1996) discuss these insufficiencies in terms of political economy, but it is at ground level that the restrictions begin to bite. Some of the restrictions to optimising research-based practice were discussed earlier in this chapter, but it is the opportunities to develop research-based practice that offer more positive ideas for devising strategies for change. In our study of practitioners' and managers' culture of research (Le May et al 1998), several existing or potential opportunities were cited (Box 8.4). Although some of these opportunities were related to individual action,

---

Box 8. 4 Opportunities to develop research-based practice

The majority of opportunities to develop research-based practice were recognised by both managers and practitioners

Organisational support
- Specific Research and Development strategy for trust or for nursing
- Enhanced links with education providers
- Funding for courses and workshops; award schemes
- Specific appointments
- Identification and support of champions for nursing

Typical quote
'Research has taken on quite strongly here because of the strategy we developed.'

New 'structures'
- Research fora
- Research awareness groups
- Proactive research/ethics committees
- Research centre
- Nursing development units

Typical quote
'It was a research awareness group and it all came about because we were sitting in the library one day talking about a course and we had a meeting the other night and it was packed with people.'

Interprofessional relationships
- Multiprofessional initiatives, e.g. guideline development
- Multidisciplinary research

Typical quote
'This is actually one way in which we are changing, we are changing the blood transfusion guidelines because we have a haematologist in our group.'

Changing individuals
- Greater uptake of continuing education
- Recognition of importance of research by individuals
- Project 2000 and degree courses increasing individual skills and knowledge

Typical quote
'Where I work now they are prepared to try.'

Reorganised NHS
- Evidence-based purchasing

Typical quote
'. . . from the view of the internal market our purchasers are expecting us to prove that we are using research-based practice.'

---

most were perceived in terms of group or organisational action. Some, such as courses on critical appraisal (Pearcey 1995), PREPP and Project 2000 (Rodgers 1994) and advisory nurses (Lacey 1994) have been cited previously. Clearly, education and information are perceived as key resources in enabling practitioners to use research more effectively (see also Chapter 6 and 7). It is essential that pressure on practitioners to change practice as a result of research are matched with an equal enthusiasm to provide them with the skills and knowledge to make this happen. There has been some evidence that managers are not totally convinced of the need for post-registration education (Caine & Kenrick 1997).

Other opportunities cited in Box 8.4 were closely linked to current governmental strategies and/or evolving professional ideologies. For example, evidence-based purchasing and enhanced links with education providers are directly associated with governmental policies, and similarly the development of Trust Research and Development strategies may be linked to the Culyer recommendations (Department of Health 1994a). Likewise, moves towards greater interdisciplinary working may be seen in terms of a developing philosophy of professional partnerships.

Evidently resources for change may 'emerge' through various routes. Sometimes they are engendered through the work of individual managers or practitioners who have the vision and persistence to ensure that potential changes are underwritten by adequate resources. In other instances it is clear that change is being driven from outside, and often this can be well financed, for example, the introduction of audit was underpinned by substantial resources. However, in both cases, either top-down or bottom-up, the danger lies in proposed changes which do not take sufficient notice of the added costs that change may bring.

MOVING FORWARD: CREATING CHANGE IN PRACTICE

This chapter has covered a substantial range of literatures and explored many aspects of change. The final section will attempt to bring together these arguments to present a viewpoint on where most capital might be gained in trying to think about and effect changes in practice which are based on evidence. At the heart of the matter lies a dilemma, for it seems that currently in health care the force for change and much of the evidence comes from the top, yet the will to change must come from the bottom. This is not to say that practitioners have nothing that they wish could be changed. On the contrary, ask any gathering of nurses and they will provide you with a fullsome list. Box 8.5 illustrates some examples of things to change which were put forward by a group of nurses attending a research utilisation workshop. The problem is that the power and wherewithal to effect change may not rest with these practitioners.

In addition, as it stands, the literature tends to take one or other approach

---

Box.8.5 Examples of things to change put forward by a group of nurses attending a research utilisation workshop

- Referral documentation
- Observation charts
- Preparation of children for painful procedures
- Staff awareness of MRSA screening
- Rotational shift pattern
- Length of stay for children on ENT wards
- Managers' views of nursing
- Admission of patients for elective surgery
- Amalgamation of consultants' ward rounds
- Role of unqualified staff
- Size of training budget
- Intransigence of educators

---

to change, either top-down, usually based on linear rational models, or bottom-up, based on ideas about empowerment and sharing. But in reality it is quite difficult to disentangle these two approaches. For example, where does the 'top' start? How many people can you practically include in your consultations when planning to make changes? What happens when you cannot reach a consensus? There is evidence that consensual agreements tend to be quite weak and general in their recommendations simply because there is only a certain number of issues on which agreement can be reached.

Despite these difficulties, common sense and experience tell us that real and sustainable change rarely occurs unless there is solid commitment from those who are expected to change. This commitment must, however, act at two levels, with both a confidence in the actual evidence on which people are supposed to act, and an alignment with the ideal behind it. It is hardly surprising, then, that both doctors and nurses are hostile to the evidence-based movement since they perceive the evidence as entirely based on research (their intuitive skills being largely discounted) and framed within a governmental ideal which they fear will threaten patient care in the drive for cost containment in the guise of efficiency and effectiveness. It would seem, then, that a bottom-up approach to change might pay greater dividends. However, the problem with bottom-up or participative change is that it often lacks sophistication in its failure to recognise both the wider effects that it may wreak, and the way in which these same issues impinge on its success.

The bottom-up approach must be more firmly embedded in a full appreciation of both the micro and macro level factors which may affect change. In other words, it is not sufficient to plan changes at, say, the level of interaction between client and nurse, without also considering the wider issues that may affect whether such change may occur, and equally how such change may in its turn affect wider issues of policy and economy. Some of the examples of desired changes in Box 8.4 would clearly involve several groups of practitioners and would have wide implications for the organisation if they were introduced.

Our change strategies must be 'informed' in the widest sense. However, as things currently stand, nursing and the professions allied to medicine must struggle to achieve this ideal because of their subordinated position and consequential lack of resources and influence. This lack does not just relate to physical items, or even numbers of staff, but to a 'capital' of skills and knowledge which is legitimised within wider society and on which nursing would then rest its power base. As Ford & Walsh (1994 p 45), drawing on the work of Friere (1985) note, domination is not just about obvious discrepancies but also 'the way ideology combines with power structures and also technology to produce types of knowledge, patterns of relationship and other cultural manifestations that operate actively to silence people'. Part of our project must, then, include a strategy to either change the current status quo in the health service hierarchy, or at least raise the issue of nursing's subordination, and the effect that it has, into the collective consciousness.

These ideas rest on the assumption that knowledge formation requires a context of equality. Thus knowledge construction in its broadest sense must rest on the existence of material and social conditions that promote freedom and equality (Nielsen 1990). As nurses of every grade and clinical speciality are aware, this state of equality does not hold true for the current culture within the NHS. The first stage of moving towards a more equitable culture must be for nurses of every level to gain a more insightful understanding of the context and implication of their subordination. Helpful here will be research emanating from critical theory and feminist perspectives which strives to identify the obstacles that distort or limit the freedom of subordinated groups.

Earlier we discussed the idea of standpoint epistemology, i.e. the idea that where you 'stand' influences what you know and how you come to know it. Thus groups such as nursing may have a more comprehensive and insightful view of NHS culture simply as a result of their particular position. We need to 'know' about doctoring for our survival as nurses, but we also 'know' about nursing in ways in which the medical profession does not. Strong & Robinson (1990), in their study of nursing following the introduction of general management into the NHS, discuss how doctors and managers were profoundly ignorant of prominent researchers and leaders in nursing. Standpoint epistemology can also be developed further through the notion of 'fusion of horizons' (Gadamer 1976). This is in fact a simple concept and relates to how each of us has a 'horizon': a certain range to our values and the stances that we take on certain matters. 'Fusion' suggests that whilst holding this stance we can explore and be open to other standpoints which may then enrich and enlarge our own ways of thinking and knowing. Through clashing with other opposing cultures, a fusion of horizons may occur. A practical example of this is provided by McPhelim & Sarvesvaran (1997): a clinical nurse specialist and a medical registrar respectively, who discuss their relationship and its impact on the care of people with lung cancer. As Sarvesvaran notes, 'I don't get sensitive about him stepping on my toes and nor does he' (p 40).

But this is starting to sound very theoretical again, when something more practical was promised. However, these ideas can be put into practice, and at an individual level many nurses are beginning to think in this way through their adoption of reflective practice. However, the project for change needs more then reflective practice enacted at the level of the nurse–client relationship. Nursing needs a critical perspective to change which incorporates reflective practice in the wider notion of conscientization. Another bit of jargon, but this stems from the work of Friere (1985) and simply relates to critical participation in transforming acts. Nursing must become conscious to itself and the influences on it. Friere's approach to change thus incorporates not only reflective practice, but also dialogue and liberation (Friere 1994). Through consciousness raising, one comes to see one's own self through the reconstruction of one's own self-formative processes (Thompson 1987). In this way, one may reflect on how the self has been fashioned through the influence of coercive power relations.

Boyce (1996), in a discussion of being a change agent, proposes that consciousness precedes individual change and dialogue precedes collective change. Drawing on her own practical experience, she explains how theory informed her practice. In her everyday work she utilises a cycle of consciousness, practice and reflective practice to engender both individual and collective change. She states that as an individual she becomes 'conscious' of the influence of her environment and aware of her actions. In 'practice' she assesses the level of skills and identifies those that will increase her effectiveness. 'Reflective practice' involves evaluating and reflecting on the results of her practice before engaging in practice again. She explains how this process must also function at an organisational level. Thus organisations must become 'conscious' of the factors – political, economic, environmental, etc. – which impinge upon them and assess how this filters down through the organisation to affect individuals and groups within it. 'Practice' at this level, according to Boyce, equates with skills needs analysis and the provision of training opportunities. Finally, 'reflective practice' is accomplished through organisational learning. This latter includes becoming aware of individuals, group processes and systems, constructing alternative actions to move towards shared goals, and enacting and evaluating these actions.

This final section has offered neither any definitive answers, nor any absolute guidelines for practice; no protocols to ensure that the next time you attempt to change things, everything will go like clockwork. What it does do is highlight some of the major dilemmas and offer some tentative ideas about the sorts of things that need to be considered when change is proposed. Hopefully it provides a rounded view, a stance which suggests that you don't take stances. Rather, in being sensitised to the theoretical issues involved, yet steeped in the everyday contingencies of practice, it is proposed that you forge an informed but meaningful approach to change: an approach that is consistent not only with your beliefs and those of your clients, but which also recognises the pragmatics of providing the most effective nursing care in today's NHS. Change is about examining your own individual practice, but it is also much more than this. It is about creating an environment where change is not perceived (as is currently the case) as another imposition from above, an irritation, yet another attempt to undermine expert practice. This will only come through a consciousness-raising exercise and a more free and equal dialogue between the different groups involved in health care provision. Sustained change can only be created through dialogue, reflective practice and liberation. As Boyce (1996 p 62) comments, '...the way in which practice occurs in an organisation is informed by how consciousness is occurring. Practice without consciousness reinforces the status quo. An enacted commitment to collective consciousness at each level of the organisation influences the conversations about needed change and individual and organisational learning'.

9

Implementing research: the practice

Trudi James   Pam Smith

INTRODUCTION

In this chapter we examine the nature of evidence, the philosophy and methods that underpin its production and its relationship to practice. We draw initially on the experiences of undertaking a research study to explore evidence in community nursing (the EECN Project) to illustrate the complex ways in which research is embedded in nurses' consciousness and interwoven into practice. We argue that the philosophy and methods used in the project, which were inspired by social, rather than biomedical, science, were more appropriate for revealing the diversity and sophistication of nurses' knowledge and practice. Following Luker & Kenrick (1992 p 463), we show that 'the distinction between scientific and experiential knowledge is an artificial one' which serves to perpetuate the divide between nursing practice and nursing research. The EECN Project and four case studies of practice developments based on research are presented. The case studies illustrate the realities of attempting to implement research in everyday practice. In the final section of the chapter we discuss the interface between the micro (project examples) and the macro (local, regional and national contexts) which both enhances and hinders the dissemination and implementation of research and the development of practice. Key issues here are: the power relations between nurses, doctors, managers and users; the impact of the contract culture and the internal market on research and professional practice; the rate of change associated with the recent reorganisation of health care; and the education of health care professionals.

Presenting research as an easily identifiable and accessible commodity just waiting to be put into practice is a notion that has been challenged by many nurses and researchers alike. Numerous barriers to the implementation of research have been documented. Some of these barriers and different approaches to creating change in practice are addressed in Chapters 4 and 8, whilst Chapter 5 specifically examines barriers to dissemination. The theoretical approaches to implementation and evidence for their effectiveness may be found in Chapter 1. Our chapter will add another dimension by showing how health care practitioners use research by providing examples of practice developments based on research. These projects have been chosen because they illustrate the realities of attempting to implement research in everyday practice.

The complex ways in which research is embedded in nurses' consciousness and becomes interwoven with other aspects of their practice, such as experience and intuition, is a process that is poorly understood. We argue that this process frequently goes unrecognised not only by nurses themselves, but also by their managers and influential others, such as chief executives of health authorities and trusts. The result has been an undervaluing of nurses' ability to utilise research in practice. We argue that one reason for the apparent 'failure' of nurses to implement research findings – so often reported in research studies – may be a reflection of the limitations of a biomedical conceptualisation of what constitutes evidence for implementation, and of the limitations of the methods utilised to conduct biomedical research (see Boxes 2.1 and 8.1). Traditionally, nursing research has been dominated by biomedical research designs which fail to reveal the diversity and sophistication of nursing's knowledge base.

EVIDENCE FOR PRACTICE

What constitutes evidence-based practice? Leading proponents of evidence-based medicine, Sackett et al (1996 p 71), consider it to be the integration of individual clinical expertise with the best available external evidence from systematic review. They also acknowledge the 'proficiency and judgment' that can result from clinical experience and practice and see it as incorporating ' ... the more thoughtful identification and compassionate use of individual patients' predicaments, rights and preferences in making clinical decisions about their care'.

The movement towards evidence-based medical and nursing care appears to have focused far more on systematic reviews and less on clinical expertise, situational knowledge and the rights and preferences of patients. The importance of systematic reviews of the literature should not be under-emphasised (see Chapter 6), particularly as there is a need to identify those areas of nursing research where a considerable body of knowledge has been accumulated and is in need of review. The existence of contradictory findings can be a source of confusion for nurses looking to the literature for answers and ways forward in the provision of care. Systematic reviews can help us to practice in ways that are underpinned by sound appraisals of the available research evidence. However, Sackett et al (1997 p 4) in relation to evidence-based medicine, warn us that we should be wary of the use of such systematic reviews as ' ... slavish, cook-book approaches to individual patient care'. This danger exists for nursing too, in its attempts to pursue the goal of evidence-based nursing practice (see also the arguments in Chapter 2).

Medical journals appear more likely than nursing journals to contain research framed by positivism (see Box 8.1), with reports of randomised controlled trials (RCTs) and follow-up studies of patients investigating a particular disease, diagnostic test or therapy. We would suggest that in the pursuit of evidence-based nursing practice, we heed Sackett's advice concerning the potential for over-reliance on systematic reviews and take it one step further.

As a result of the interpretive orientation of much current nursing research, the nature of the body of knowledge contained within it varies considerably from medicine. The recognition that major changes have occurred in the way that knowledge is produced is apparent in a recent text written by an interdisciplinary group of authors (Gibbons et al 1994). They describe the shift from the conventional scientific mode of knowledge production to a new mode that is 'non-linear' in that it does not depend on the testing of hypotheses and theory. This new mode of knowledge production values reflexivity, transdisciplinarity and difference: familiar concepts in the world of nursing research. It draws on a range of settings, sources and processes to produce it. It also supports a research agenda that we propose for nursing, which is committed to exploring and legitimating different knowledge forms (see also Chapter 3).

Evidence for nursing should reflect the different orientation of nursing practice and research. This does not mean rejecting all that has been learnt through the use of positivist science. Some of the principles that lead to rigour in research are important. It is possible to present a very partial view (accepting that all views describe only part of the whole anyway) under the guise of research. The integration of subjectivity does not mean that the researcher's view 'rules OK'. The challenge is to integrate the subjective with the objective in a way which moves beyond the futility of the subjectivity/objectivity divide. Nurse researchers who have popularised the use of triangulation, for example, have, in their use of multiple sources of data, methods and theoretical schemes, adopted an interpretive approach designed to give an in-depth understanding of the phenomena under study. They have sought to establish a 'negotiated reality' of the research setting. This is illustrated by the following quotation in which Denzin (1989 p 235), who popularised the use of triangulation amongst sociologists, states: 'Methods are like the kaleidoscope, depending on how they are approached, held, and acted toward, different observations will be revealed. This is not to imply that reality has the shifting qualities of the coloured prism, but that it too is an object that moves and that will not permit one interpretation to be stamped upon it'.

All perspectives dangle from each person's personal constructs. Views, truths and conceptions of the 'real' world, therefore, can never be wholly ripped away from the people who experience them. In determining what constitutes evidence for nursing, dangers to be avoided include: context stripping; producing results following the conventional scientific model which simplify the world in order to make it understandable; withdrawing as a researcher into an assumed position of neutrality; and presenting an idiosyncratic perspective as 'the reality'. The evidence we use to guide our practice needs to be dynamic, to reflect multiple realities and nurses' use of intuition and experience. It requires an emphasis on the relational nature of nursing and the varying contexts and values that shape it. We need to give a high priority to reviewing and developing research which explores the proficiency and judgment embedded in the clinical experience of nurses. At the same time, reviews of research are required which reveal the best possible ways of incorporating patients' predicaments, rights and preferences into our practice.

If we follow the lead of medicine where the systematic review of RCTs has been emblazoned with the gold standard, complex issues and vast bodies of expertise in nursing could be overlooked. It has been recognised for some time within sociology that language is important in constituting social order and reality (Atkinson 1990). The language used to describe the RCT research environment, for example as 'the gold standard', conjures up a somewhat uncomfortable vision of a soldier – for which, read doctor in shining armour brandishing a flag. This vision carries with it the imagery of battle: one that is 'man-made', and well suited to the language that medicine has traditionally used with regard to fighting disease. Standards are for excellence but they also denote taking up arms, leading the way into battle. We do not need to gird ourselves with a belt full of cartridges as the title of the evidence-based health care journal *Bandolier* suggests, so that we have ammunition/'magic bullets' to fire at people. Our path in nursing, whilst recognising the value of RCTs, should be one that enables us to embrace broader concepts such as excellence in nursing practice as it contributes to effectiveness (A Pearson, unpublished work, 1997), even if the route is less well travelled. Rather than falling in line behind medicine's banner, nurses can decide to fly a different flag – one that will tell us more about the highly valued human component of work, our relationships with patients, the centrality of reclaiming a passion for caring in nursing and nursing research (Cotter & Smith 1998), and the concerns that patients themselves have. In fact it would be surprising if medicine itself would not find such an approach useful (see Cochrane 1972 pp 94–95). Certainly some doctors have raised queries about the current model of evidence-based practice (Jenkins 1991). The nursing research literature abounds with findings that show us the value of such concepts for nurses and their patients and clients. However, it is important to question the extent to which nurses have been influenced by, and have influenced, this body of research. Nevertheless, the fact that a literature exists which describes such beliefs and values about nursing practice should give us a clue to the way forward.

To illustrate our points about nurses' embedded knowledge and non-conscious (taken here to mean being unaware of, or not recognising) approaches to research implementation, we discuss here a project that one of the authors (Trudi) was involved in. We reflect on the project to explore the use of evidence in community nursing practice and reveal ways in which evidence was integrated into the process of a variety of different community nurses' work. The key words here are 'evidence', 'integrated' and 'process'. The nature of evidence in nursing, its integration into practice and the process of its implementation will be considered with reference to the position of nurses vis-a-vis their power in the medical and nursing hierarchy, the invisibility of core elements of their practice and the degree to which users are involved in making decisions about the care they receive.

THE EXPLORING EVIDENCE IN COMMUNITY NURSING (EECN) PROJECT

The EECN project focused on the nature and use of evidence and its implementation in community nursing, rather than practice development and research implementation per se. However, the findings have something to say about what constitutes evidence for effective practice, and the current predominance of certain types of evidence over others. The study design and methods also illustrate that exploring the issue of evidence for, and in, nursing practice from a psychosocial rather than a biomedical perspective, provides us with different meanings and interpretations. Some of these are consonant with the conventional scientific construction of evidence and others extend beyond the horizons of biomedicine. Our research revealed that, a little like an iceberg, much of the evidence that nurses use that contributes to the effectiveness of their practice is not easily discernible, yet it affects the likely outcomes for patients/clients in very tangible ways.

In comparison to the work of nurses in inpatient settings, community nursing is under-researched. The findings from one key study (Luker & Kenrick 1992 p 464) exploring the sources of influence on the clinical decisions of community nurses suggest that ' ... it is conceivable that community nurses are being exposed to research findings, which have been reclassified as nursing knowledge, and are therefore not aware of the extent to which research informs their practice'. They conclude that work is required to explore the ways in which this reclassification occurs and research is integrated into the nursing knowledge base. The results of the EECN Project shed some light on this process of integration and offer an insight into the evidence that community nurses use to inform their practice.

Funded by North Thames Regional Health Authority and conducted in Camden and Islington, and Tower Hamlets Community Trusts, this study used an eclectic multi-method approach involving a questionnaire, semi-structured interviews, focus groups and non-participant observation. The research proposal was formulated by Valerie Buxton, a part-time lecturer in primary health care at UCL Medical School, with the support of the Directors of Nursing Services in both trusts and the Director of Research and Health Promotion in Camden and Islington. Academic and clinical links were already forged to some extent, aided by the fact that the four people involved in the project had all previously worked in one or both trusts in clinical or administrative roles. The two main aims of the project were:

1. to consider the nature of evidence within community nursing practice
2. to identify the factors that influence the use of evidence in community nursing practice.

Two hundred and twenty-three community nurses completed the questionnaire; 56 interviews were conducted with nurse managers and others in senior positions whose remit included developing/supporting the use of research in practice; and individual interviews and focus groups were carried out with 55 nurses who were willing to explore their use of research and other evidence through the device of a family scenario. The scenario comprised a family tree with a brief outline of the health problems of each family member. Sixteen community nurses allowed us to observe their practice. The observation sessions were followed by interviews where field notes were checked with the nurses involved to enhance consistency/dependability and credibility, and to facilitate a deeper understanding of the ways in which evidence was utilised in the health care encounters that we observed (Hall & Stevens 1991). Our aim was to adequately reflect the complexity of the events being observed, taking account of the contexts of participants' lives.

We would support Luker & Kenrick's (1992) contention that questions need to be raised about the perpetuation of the divide between nursing practice and nursing research. Both endeavours (if we accept the need to situate the nurse researcher, her or his values, subjectivity and nursing experience in the research process) incorporate elements of the other. That is, the nurse researcher brings elements of her or his knowledge of practice to bear upon the study, and the nurse practitioner incorporates elements of research into her or his work. Both processes require far more elucidation: neither role/job is necessarily superior to the other. This 'interweaving' of practice and research was apparent in the data generated in the EECN Project. From analysis of the interviews, focus groups and participant observation, it became clear that nurses were drawing upon a sophisticated matrix of evidence in order to enhance patient care.

The process of integration

The findings, particularly from the observational phase of the EECN Project showed that nurses use evidence derived from a number of different sources. One such source appears to have its origins in what Karen

Davies (1990) has called a 'nurturing rationality', that is, an orientation to others that takes their needs and reality into account. Davies maintains that this orientation is associated with women's care work, and forms an integral part of their consciousness. Observing nurses' practice revealed for Trudi that the centrality of this response to human need and the importance of developing and maintaining relationships acted as both sources of evidence for nurses to draw upon, and ways of utilising embedded research knowledge.

Whilst evidence of the use of scientific research was apparent in the health care encounters observed, the use of ethical, personal and intuitive knowledge was also reflected. Morse et al (1994) have demonstrated the ability of nurses to sense the needs and conditions of their patients as part of the humanistic dimension of nursing. Intuition, inference, emotional empathy, 'knowing', counter-transference, compathy and embodiment are concepts that she uses to describe 'sensing' patient needs. Morse et al (1994 p 273) define compathy as 'the response that occurs when a person observes physical distress/suffering in another person, and the observer experiences similar distress or symptoms'. Observational data from the EECN Project revealed that nurses' ability to sense patients' needs informed their decision making, acting as what we have called 'feeling' evidence.

On the surface it was not always apparent what evidence was being used to make decisions about patient care. Exploring this in more depth with nurses, several features were identifiable. These were: knowledge of the individual patients and their ways of 'seeing'; information gathered about likely behaviour from previous encounters with individual patients; visual and other sensory evidence; the effects of decisions made in the past in relation to individual patients; and the nurses' own accumulated clinical and life experiences. These findings are not dissimilar to research on the nature of intuition carried out by Easen & Wilcockson (1996 p 672). They argue that a number of different rational components contribute to the existence of an intuitive process discernible in both nursing and teaching. They state:

Of primary importance is a sound, relevant knowledge base and the ability to recognise patterns in the presenting problem. Such pattern recognition is rooted in past decision-making and experience and is essential for this linking of similar past events to the present. Embedded within the intuiter's performance is implicit thinking and the use of the professional's 'know-how' ... with the passing of time, some of this knowledge may become tacit.

Intuition may be equated with magic, myth or tradition and is not necessarily perceived as unscientific or without worth. In the words of one district nurse, speaking about the ways in which we devalue the intrinsic aspects of our work, 'Sometimes tradition can be evidence-based as well, but it's just that someone hasn't sat down and thought about it logically or looked at it scientifically'. One example of this emerged during an interview with a health visitor who stated that throughout the 20 years that she had been practising she had purposefully visited women with post-natal depression on a weekly basis. She had searched for 'scientific' evidence of the effectiveness of this approach in order to convince her managers of the positive outcomes of this practice that she was witnessing. Only in more recent years has such evidence emerged.

Another example of the need for practice-based research was offered by an Asian health visitor who commented that research on the Bangladeshi population tended to focus largely on those in lower socio-economic groups. She pointed out that the original immigrants from Bangladesh were predominantly working class, but that in recent years middle class families had come to the UK. Yet research was failing to relate to this changing population and persisted in representing people from Bangladesh as impoverished and educationally inferior. There were many such examples apparent in our interview data which revealed that nurses know what questions to ask, but are not always enabled to ask them or to make their voices heard.

Research can lag behind practice and may not adequately reflect the changing world in which we live and work. Paying attention to and evaluating what is valuable to patients and nurses about the caring we do may just provide the kinds of evidence we need, which are not just about proving our effectiveness but also about showing that what people feel and have to say really matters. The following four case studies provide examples of practice developments based on research where the desire to deliver effective care appeared to be part of a broader commitment to practice in ways which are humane and compassionate, emphasising our connectedness with one another. Individuals were approached to share their experiences of practice development and their feelings about these with us in an informal interview. Projects were selected to provide examples from both inpatient and community settings. Inter- and multidisciplinary working are common features in the case studies. We also endeavoured to elicit the 'behind the scenes' factors likely to contribute to, or hinder, successful research implementation that are not so widely shared in published reports of research.

CASE STUDY 1: THE UTILISATION OF RESEARCH IN PRACTICE – A STRATEGY FOR CHANGE

The Nursing Research and Practice Development Unit at St James's and Seacroft University Hospitals was established in 1992 to promote the use of research in practice. Michelle Briggs joined the team that year as a research and development practitioner with an interest in the management of pain gained during her experience of working in the field of trauma orthopaedics.

The Unit was small, so a strategy was developed which focused on using research in practice, concentrating on four key themes: wound care; pressure sore prevention; pain; and documentation. The strategy development was led by Jane Nixon (Head of the Unit) and involved widespread consultation with staff across the trust. The choice of themes were influenced by the following factors:

- their relevance to the majority of specialities within the trust
- the existence of evidence of good multidisciplinary support
- they constituted areas where nursing greatly contributed to the overall quality of care
- they constituted a major resource issue both locally and nationally
- the research and development practitioner had an academic interest in the theme
- they built on existing development work within the trust.

At the time of Michelle's appointment, a working group concerned with pain management (the Acute Pain Service Working Group) had been established by a consultant anaesthetist with a particular interest in the subject. This group was multidisciplinary and had representatives from anaesthetics, general surgery, the chronic pain team, physiotherapy, pharmacy and the palliative care team. However, despite this there was no regular nursing input, and Michelle therefore offered to participate in the steering group – a move which was welcomed by the consultant concerned. Michelle then set up an acute pain nursing working group whose views she could feed into the steering group. Between 30 and 40 nurses of all grades were involved in this group. The meetings were always well attended because, Michelle believes, the nurses were fully aware of what they wanted to achieve in the area of pain management, but there had never been a mechanism in place through which their voices could be heard. With the development of the Unit with its research and practice development strategy and the initiation of the acute pain nursing working group, that mechanism was now in place. A process was being facilitated that would enable change to occur (see Chapter 8 on factors that affect change).

Practitioners' desire to improve pain management was supported in the literature by research findings which indicated that there was a need to challenge traditional attitudes to postoperative pain, to improve staff education, to assess and record pain systematically and to continue to appraise that activity. Subsequently a baseline audit was undertaken to:

1. ascertain the levels of pain that patients were experiencing postoperatively
2. assess the clinical practice relating to acute pain using an audit framework.

The findings indicated poor pain assessment, under-utilisation of patient-controlled analgesia and epidural pain relief, and inadequate provision of information to patients about pain. As a result of this audit and its presentation to the acute pain groups, the following recommendations for practice were agreed:

- the provision of multidisciplinary guidelines on acute pain assessment and management
- implementation of a pain assessment system for all patients
- optimising the use of patient-controlled analgesia by centralising the relevant pumps within the post-anaesthetic care unit and developing the role of nurses in that unit
- organisation of the multidisciplinary education programme
- provision of more information for patients about pain
- the development of a network with an acute pain link nurse on each ward within the surgical specialities with a responsibility for implementing pain assessment, evaluation and improved documentation.

The development of these recommendations was seen very much as a collaborative process, whereby interested parties were given adequate opportunities to contribute to the content and format of proposals. The recommendations provided a framework to change practice, and a repeat audit was undertaken to assess how far the recommendations had been implemented. The repeat audit revealed that pain assessment and documentation had improved dramatically, patient-controlled analgesia pumps were being more efficiently used due to an increase in their availability at the point of need, and there had also been an increase in the amount of information that patients received.

However, the audit team was unable to demonstrate a reduction in patients' pain scores as a result of these changes. This may have been because the audit method focused mainly on process issues (e.g. whether a pain score was documented) rather than outcomes. In addition, the pain rating instrument that was used was a five-point verbal rating scale which may not have been sensitive enough to detect pre- and post-intervention differences in the small groups included. Furthermore, pain outcomes are affected by numerous multidisciplinary inputs, and it is difficult to control all the variables that may affect these outcomes within the resources of an audit project. Hence the audit demonstrated improved quality and efficient use of resources, but the effectiveness of the changes could not be assessed using this method.

One particular limitation highlighted by the reaudit was the lack of uptake of the recommendations at night. So Michelle secured funding from the Northern and Yorkshire region in collaboration with Dr Jose Closs (who led the research team) to evaluate the effectiveness of specific interventions to improve pain management at night based on the principles outlined in the guidelines. This generated an opportunity for a research secondment for another member of staff, Viv Everitt. Viv's experience and advice enabled the development and adaptation of the recommendations into a format more suitable for use at night.

A number of other supportive factors were influential in improving the use of research evidence in acute pain practice. A clear strategy for change and managerial support from the chief nursing officer and divisional nurse managers had contributed to the success of the project. They ensured that it had a high profile and provided the necessary time for link nurse education, audit workshops, presentations at sisters' meetings, and attendance at the acute pain nursing working group. The divisional nurse manager for theatres fully supported the baseline audit data collection by the full-time release of a member of staff for 1 month, and successfully negotiated dedicated acute pain nursing support within the post-anaesthetic care unit. Also of importance was the educational support provided to Michelle and the study of the subject area at master's level at Leeds Metropolitan University. This example of clinical development work echoes the crucial importance of managerial support which is also discussed in Chapter 7 in relation to Project 2000 students, and in Chapter 8 in relation to change management.

A similar strategy to facilitate research utilisation was employed for the other practice development themes. In particular, the use of link nurses from each of the clinical areas who were responsible for local implementation was particularly effective at the implementation stage. A job description was compiled for the acute pain, pressure sore and wound care link nurses who were supported by the lead research and development practitioner in a reflective process which involved reviewing progress and addressing any problems as they arose. The outcome of this exercise was very positive. In relation to wound management, providing guidelines, education via the link nurses and a structured framework of assessment raised the standards of documentation of wound management and resulted in savings through the rationalisation of wound care products. With regard to the implementation of the pressure sore care policy, major cost savings were achieved, the provision of pressure-relieving equipment was increased, and savings were made. Jane then negotiated for these savings to be utilised to purchase equipment required for safe handling practice.

And so the Unit has moved on to other practice development themes. The team members are currently focusing on nutritional care, continence, evidence-based criteria for the selection of clinical products, and reviewing practice in relation to key components of a philosophy of nursing identified as: beliefs, religion and customs; privacy and dignity; and the promotion of choice and health.

In summary, fundamental to the success of the work of the Unit are a number of factors which are broadly applicable in the pursuit of research implementation. Structural issues require careful assessment and handling;

wide consultation is necessary, with the involvement of all levels of staff within the organisation. A mechanism needs to be developed for people to be heard and to get involved. Flexibility helps, as people bring to the various projects different ways of working and different approaches. Regular contact with other health care practitioners is also needed to build a relationship that can enable multidisciplinary working. Care in selecting practice development themes is also required. An in-depth understanding of subject areas at degree and postgraduate levels ensures credibility across specialities and disciplines, and enables the translation of a broad literature into guidelines that have practical application. Implementing a piece of research before careful assessment of its suitability and likely application, and without an understanding of the resulting organisational and practical problems that may arise may cause an initiative to break down very quickly.

A great deal has been achieved at the Nursing Research and Practice Development Unit in the past 5 years. The future challenges include:

- developing a core group of nurses with advanced skills to appraise research and synthesise its findings into guidance for practice
- developing other methods of supporting clinicians to change their practice
- using systematic reviews which summarise available research on the effectiveness of specific interventions (see Chapter 6).

CASE STUDY 2: DEVELOPMENT OF A NURSING STRATEGY FOR RESEARCH AND DISSEMINATION IN AN NHS TRUST

Jackie Solomon is Senior Nurse for Research and Development in Bolton Hospitals NHS Trust. In a telephone interview she described how a nursing strategy for research and development was developed within the Acute Hospitals Trust. The work began in 1993 following the publication of the Department of Health *Report of the Task Force on the Strategy for Research in Nursing, Midwifery and Health Visiting* (Department of Health 1993b). To explore the implications for practice arising from this document, a working group involving senior nurses in the trust and educationalists was set up. A SWOT (strengths, weaknesses, opportunities, threats) analysis revealed research to be small-scale and fragmented in the trust, and although there were pockets of interested and committed staff, there was a general lack of research appreciation and awareness amongst nurses with little sharing of ideas, poor communication and lots of duplication. It was also evident that there was no structure to support research and dissemination, although resources did exist, such as access to information technology and an on-site library in the College of Nursing. Other strengths were identified in the behaviour of Project 2000 students, who were asking questions of ward staff and acting as a stimulus. Using the information gained from this analysis, the group utilised the four priority areas in the *Report of the Task Force on the Strategy for Research in Nursing, Midwifery and Health Visiting* (Department of Health 1993b): dissemination; implementation; education and training; and careers to identify aims related to each of these issues. Subsequently a structure and way of working began to emerge which, in the following 4 years (it takes time), has stimulated a more positive research culture.

What specific attributes and factors then, contributed to the creation of this culture? With the nursing strategy in place, a research and development forum was instigated. This acted as a focus for the research and development coordinators from each of the directorates to share ideas and innovations. For example, a particular topic might be selected such as preoperative fasting. This would involve the general surgical, anaesthetic, theatre, and specialist surgery directorates. Their aim would be to evaluate current research and its application to practice, facilitate its dissemination and identify future research priorities. Throughout this process, the training and development needs of staff were also being determined. Following the publication of the research and development strategy, one of the first training and development initiatives was a 4-day workshop: 'Effective utilisation of research' organised by the Foundation of Nursing Studies. Both managers and practitioners attended this workshop.

To provide education and training for clinical staff to develop their research awareness, Jackie worked with a lecturer from Salford University to create a 6-day in-house course running 1 day a month over 6 months. She was particularly concerned with enabling staff to attend who had had little exposure to research in their pre- or post-registration education. The success of the course has resulted in plans to open it up to other professional groups such as occupational therapists, podiatrists and physiotherapists, and a move to seek accreditation through Salford University. Underpinning the course are the beliefs that it should be of relevance to nurses' clinical practice, be of interest and of help to them, and be rooted in their everyday working lives. Embodied in this approach is a pragmatism that recognises that simply giving information to nurses is not enough. They need to acquire the confidence to identify how the knowledge they have gained can meaningfully be applied in an area of their practice in collaboration with colleagues and managers. The specific objectives of the course were therefore designed to enable participants to:

- describe the research process
- recognise different approaches to, and ways of, utilising research
- undertake a literature search in relation to a specific area of practice

- describe local and national initiatives in relation to research and dissemination
- identify professional and ethical implications of research practice
- present an action plan of how an aspect of research-based practice could be developed within their own field.

During the course, participants are expected to keep a reflective diary, and to reflect on what is research-based in their practice. This is discussed with staff on the ward and with their mentor. Subsequently they bring these reflections and outcomes of the discussions with their colleagues to the study days. On the final day of the course, with nurse managers present, students present their action plans.

Keeping research alive in the trust is also achieved by a research interest group for staff with different levels of research expertise which meets every 2 months. It operates as a networking event, a forum for sharing information and experiences of doing research, and as a means of meeting external researchers, who are invited in as key speakers. Workshops are also available for practitioners to develop skills in critical appraisal of research evidence. These are run by a research fellow from Salford University and are multidisciplinary, drawing senior and junior nursing and medical staff together. The skills developed in these workshops can be further employed in the journal club. Here a research fellow and a statistician support staff in reviewing research papers during a lunchtime session that lasts for 90 minutes.

One of the pleasing and surprising outcomes of the emergence of a more positive research culture in the trust was the escalation of a plan for a local area research workshop in 1996 into a national research conference. It was followed in 1997 by a second such event. Both conferences were organised with the help of the Foundation of Nursing Studies, whose support was crucial to their success. As the conferences were run locally, nurses submitted abstracts, some of which were selected. Coaching and support were then offered to enable them to take part with confidence. Other nurses from the trust who attended saw their colleagues, staff nurses and sisters, giving papers and began to think 'I could do this too'. At the time we spoke to Jackie, at least 6 nurses were preparing to speak at conferences in the coming 3 months.

Whilst the initiatives described above provide some insight into the developmental process – the 'how' of creating a thriving research environment – as with the other projects we have described, certain less obvious factors were also influential. The process worked well where managers had an understanding of research themselves and were willing to empower their staff. Some directorates appeared to have more knowledge of research and a greater appreciation of its value. Where those with most power and authority act as 'champions' of research, the dissemination process appears to be more effective. In one such directorate, the research interest group has now become multidisciplinary and acts as a catalyst for change.

Paying attention to the cultural differences between medicine and nursing is also part of the process of implementing research successfully. Enabling medical staff to reach an understanding of the nurse's role and that their approaches to research may well differ, contributes to multidisciplinary working. Doctors' experiences of research are more likely to be grounded in clinical trials and in the need to establish scientific truth. Our interview with Jackie suggested that some nurses appear to have a different outlook, and to be asking different questions, such as:

- the evidence derived from randomised controlled trials on a particular subject is one-dimensional: what other ways are there of looking at what constitutes evidence for practice in this situation?
- what criteria should be included in a framework for critically appraising qualitative research?
- can this piece of evidence be implemented in practice, how realistic is it to try?

These differences are potential strengths, but nurses need training and education to enable them to debate this in an arena that favours a biomedical construction of evidence and clinical effectiveness. That is why Jackie is aiming to prepare nurses to take a full part in that debate, to ensure that their voices are heard, in the diverse ways outlined above. Building on the nursing strategy at a more advanced level, she is also encouraging secondment and is actively seeking opportunities for them to participate in multidisciplinary courses on evidence-based practice at the University of Central Lancashire, and working with Salford University to provide access for nurses to study at master's level. Within such a strategy, she believes the dissemination and implementation of research can be facilitated and sustained. Finally, in relating this case study to the authors, Jackie stressed the support that she had had from all the practitioners, managers and educationalists whose help and hard work had contributed to the success of the initiative that she described.

CASE STUDY 3: GETTING THE BASICS RIGHT – THE DEVELOPMENT OF NURSES' SKILLS IN ASSESSMENT AND CARE PLANNING

This project addressing the issues of assessment, care planning and evaluation was a collaborative venture between the Guy's and St Thomas' Hospital NHS Trust and the Foundation of Nursing Studies. Its aim has been to develop proactively managed nursing care. The project was part of the vision of the professional leader of nursing at the trust: Wilma MacPherson, Director of Quality and Nursing. It was brought into life through the engagement and cooperation of groups of nurses working collaboratively with the Foundation's Project Development Officer, and was transformed into practice through the leadership of the ward sister. We interviewed Caroline Alexander, the Project Development Officer involved from the Foundation, about the realities of trying to implement research of this nature in diverse inpatient settings. Many of the problems that she discusses below may be familiar to those of you who work in similar settings. Hopefully this case study will provide you with some insights into how such areas of difficulty may be best managed.

Caroline was employed on a contractual basis for one day a week initially to develop assessment, care planning and evaluation skills and documentation. However, it soon became clear that focusing solely on improving the documentation, as has been done in the past, would not necessarily effect lasting change for the better. Following an audit, she found that both nurses and teachers were using the nursing process because they felt they had to, with little understanding of why they were using it: assessment and care planning were being narrowly construed as recording admission details/data collection and describing rather than prescribing care; there was an apparent lack of patient involvement in the decision-making and evaluation process; and nurses had taken on non-nursing duties that were preventing them from nursing. It was also evident that nurses tended to plan care around medical diagnoses focusing on impairment and disability.

This was nursing at its most task-focused and reactive, in support of, and framed by, the medical model. The overall impression was one of disempowerment: nurses seemed to have lost what was essentially nursing; they felt stuck and unable to be proactive or change and were frustrated by numerous obstacles preventing them from giving nursing care.

Caroline felt that the general lack of understanding about the work that nurses do and the low value placed upon nursing contributed to the climate of reactivity and a diminished sense of responsibility for promoting the effectiveness of the documentation of the nursing process and nursing care. A culture of not questioning arising from a socialisation process reinforcing this reactivity meant that nurses were uncertain if or how they could effect change. In addition, it appeared that the care being given to patients was often completely at odds with what was written on the care plan. Nurses were not reviewing the care they were giving, as evaluation was poorly understood and therefore was not well done.

If the nursing process documentation was ever to be effectively utilised, Caroline determined that nurses required a say: no-one had asked them what their perceptions were of the situation, or what difficulties they faced, or what they wanted. Having decided on this approach, nurses were then invited to voice their concerns, with organisational as well as individual and collective responsibilities being identified for resolving those problems. Through seeking to recognise and understand the real contribution of nursing, ownership of the process of change by nurses in clinical practice was encouraged. Subsequently, attention shifted to the philosophy and fundamental principles underpinning nursing and decision making in order for them to become, 'reestablished and internalised in the minds of nurses'. In particular, nurses concentrated on the decision-making process in nursing assessment, care planning and evaluation, critically evaluating their practice and seeking ways to actively involve patients. Over 150 nurses participated in focus groups and workshops to share what they perceived to be the process and principles of nursing, focusing back on the patient as an individual rather than the tasks to be identified. Two key issues emerged:

1. the care needs of the patient must be put into the context of the patient's life and lifestyle
2. care must be proactively managed by managing the handicap, i.e. the effect of impaired function on the person's life.

An influential factor in achieving the required changes was effective ward management and leadership. The ward sister was a key figure in the implementation process who would share the vision of a more proactive approach to managing nursing care with the other staff.

In retrospect, Caroline felt that it was the developmental process itself that mattered the most. This appears to have been an evolutionary process where valuable aspects of the hierarchical structure, peer group work and individual leadership enabled articulation of what nurses could do to develop their own decision-making and care management skills. Two hundred staff have taken part in the 2-day implementation workshops over 2 years, and the principles for practice, identified in the focus groups carried out in the 10 pilot wards (a mixture of medical and surgical specialities), are now being extended to other wards.

In conveying to us for the purpose of this chapter how clinical practice was influenced and developed, it was evident that other less tangible facets relating to the relational/emotional life of the project had contributed to its success. The use of empathy, being willing to listen and reflect and taking responsibility all appear to have played a large part in the transformation to proactively managed nursing care. These characteristics can be seen to be embedded in the stories Caroline told us about significant project events. One such 'marker' was the dawning of recognition amongst nurses given time to reflect on their practice that 'We just do it (nursing)...we ignore the patients'. Their horror at the realisation that they often presumed that they knew what their patients wanted opened the door to more attuned practice in assessment and care planning. At the same time, in seeking to address the very real organisational barriers to research implementation that the nurses had identified, a concerted effort was made to deal with these at various levels. Changing the practice of individuals without addressing organisational constraints would be strategically unproductive.

For Caroline, who was contracted from an 'outside body' to improve the documentation of the nursing process in the hospital, a certain amount of resistance was anticipated. She had previously been employed as a ward sister and practice development nurse in the trust, and returning in a different role was difficult. To be accepted, she had to prove her credibility. By choosing a line of action that emphasised her beliefs that nursing is undervalued, and in seeking a role that listened to and enabled nurses' voices to be heard, it was possible to effect change. What made a difference is her identification with the position of nurses, the desire to listen and reflect, and then to promote the ability of nurses to articulate and then internalise the contribution that their work makes in health and illness care; for them to have ownership of this process and its products: more knowledgeable doers leading to better care.

Caroline's commitment to the nurses and the trust she had formerly worked in was destined to escalate the size and scope of the project, which did, however, have to continue to operate within time and budget constraints. The project and those who were, and continue to be, part of it overcame many barriers, for example: having to achieve change in a climate of frequent reorganisations; repeatedly having to prove the worth and relevance of the project; resisting the desire to 'jump on the bandwagon', uncritically adopting and putting research into practice because of the pressure to become a research-based profession; short-term funding operating within the constraints of the contract culture and the resulting restrictive effects on long-term planning and sustained development; the 'out on a limb' nature of professional development nurse posts, their lack of authority and their ambivalent place in the management power structure; and the sometimes conflicting interests of trusts, health care practitioners, patients, other stakeholders and the body for whom the management consultant/researcher works.

In summary, this project has established workshops that offer nurses the tools to start changing their own practice. From the data generated at the workshops and focus groups, a working standard for assessment, care planning and evaluation has emerged. The project has now come to a close and Caroline has withdrawn, but the trust is developing a training pack to take the initiative forward, and the workshop programme for nurses will continue following the training of workshop leaders. Constraints identified in these group meetings will continue to be addressed, and staff made aware of the outcomes to ensure that the trust is seen to be responsive and committed to the project. Although the initial aim of the project was to improve documentation, it soon became obvious that sound principles for decision making and a better understanding of the contribution of nursing to managed care were essential prerequisites to good documentation. Documentation that is user-friendly is the aim, and it is intended that staff carry out the audit process in order to facilitate improvements in the quality of nursing documentation and to take the project forward themselves.

CASE STUDY 4: THE LEG ULCER PROJECT

The Primary Care Development Unit is part of Waltham Forest Healthcare Trust Primary Health Care Directorate. It was established in January 1997, has three nurse members and has a vision of how to support and develop primary health care teams, and the nurses at their core. The aims of the Unit are:

1. to support primary health care teams towards an integrated approach in identifying, planning, coordinating and delivering care
2. to develop and implement an education and training strategy for the directorate
3. to promote research and audit within the directorate
4. to develop and implement systems for clinical supervision
5. to develop and implement a child protection strategy
6. to develop a recruitment strategy for the directorate
7. to develop and implement a primary care strategy for the directorate.

We interviewed Pam Fenner, Manager of the Primary Care Development Unit about a 2-year project initiated a short time before the unit opened. Its aim was to implement evidence-based practice in the care of patients with leg ulcers in the community – a large part of the work of district nurses in the trust. Whilst having considerable resource implications with regard to time and money, Pam described the human cost of leg ulcers in terms of the pain, reduced mobility and the restrictions they imposed on the social life of individuals affected, as 'a sea of patients' suffering'. A consultant vascular surgeon at Whipps Cross Hospital was also concerned that there was no standardisation of treatment for patients with leg ulcers, and that a myriad of different treatments were being used by district nurses. Having put together a paper reviewing the available evidence, it was clear that there was a case for change.

To find a way forward, Pam visited the community-based leg ulcer clinics established by the clinical nurse specialist at Charing Cross where they were using a standardised approach and achieving 70% healing rates at 12 weeks. The team at Charing Cross was contracted to work with Waltham Forest to implement a similar system of community clinics. Having identified a course of action and a source of expertise to draw upon, financing the project was now the major concern. In particular, the four-layer compression bandages needed as a core part of the standardised treatment were not available on FP10 prescription, i.e. funding was required.

At the time, in the wake of the Tomlinson Report (1992), London Implementation Zone money became available and the Health Authority asked them to prepare a bid. From the beginnings of an idea, through an exploratory phase to the development of an adequate proposal took approximately 6 months. A 2-year programme was envisaged which would be led by a clinical nurse specialist and would include training for staff and access to the ENB leg ulcer course (N18) run by the clinical nurse specialist from Charing Cross. Eight coordinators would be appointed to run four leg ulcer clinics following completion of the ENB course. The bid was successful and they secured funding of £180 000.

Implementation of the project was guided by a steering group. This comprised Pam as chair, a district nurse manager, a Family Health Services Authority (FHSA) locality manager, the consultant vascular surgeon, a clinic administrator, hotel services, nurse representatives and a general practitioner. The clinical nurse specialist was appointed and the process of setting up the teams began. The coordinators were going to be the major change agents and were perceived to be vitally important. Care was taken to establish how potential appointees would manage change, cope with conflict, and communicate to take the new service forward.

The project was met with a degree of resistance. Some district nurses felt that it would impose on their right to make an assessment, and they showed a great attachment to the treatments they were currently using. Company representatives proved another stumbling block, since nurses were keen to try various other products that they were marketing. Action was taken that banned all representatives of dressing companies from calling at health centres in order to counteract the problem and promote the standardised approach being recommended. At the same time a baseline audit of local practice carried out by Charing Cross revealed the tremendous variety of leg ulcer treatments being provided by nurses, their cost, the time spent on them and the slow rates of healing. Nurses recognised that here was evidence of the need for change. However, the project was not just about cost and compression bandages, but about a whole way of managing leg ulcers. As well as offering patients a standardised, evidence-based treatment, bringing them by ambulance to the clinics became a social occasion. Tea and coffee were provided and people started to get to know one another. Nurses noticed that clients were dressing up to come to the clinics, some of the women wore hats, and many appeared to look forward to the visit as though it were a social occasion. We would argue that these are important outcome measures of effectiveness. Attendance rates were high. Word spread through the community and people living in a neighbouring area wrote to their local MP, demanding the same facilities from their health authority. The neighbouring trust went through a similar process and secured funding to establish leg ulcer clinics for their local population. This was a further indication of effective implementation, in that it empowered members of the community to take action that resulted in access to better and more equitable services. There were benefits too for auxiliary nurses, as they took advantage of the accreditation towards the National Vocational Qualification (NVQ) that the experience in the clinics afforded them: a tangible educational outcome. The programme also brought community nurses and hospital-based medical and nursing staff closer together. The clinical nurse specialist worked collaboratively with the consultant vascular surgeon in the hospital-based leg ulcer clinic and formed a point of contact for inpatient staff. The clinic coordinators and district nurses received training, and having implemented treatment with the four-layer compression bandage, achieved a healing rate of over 70% at 12 weeks. General practitioners were delighted with this outcome and with the added bonus of no longer having to pay for the variety of lotions and dressings that nurses had previously used. This project had many positive developmental outcomes that would not be reflected using the limited measures of effectiveness contained within traditional models for evaluating successful implementation of research.

However, a shadow hangs over the project. It was envisaged that, given the research evidence for the effectiveness of four-layer compression bandages, they would be offered free to patients on FP10. As yet the bandages are not available on prescription, and when the project money ran out, the health authority was not able to fund the treatment separately. The money had to come out of normal budgets. The reality is that £35 000 per year to cover the cost of the bandages and £10 000 for the ambulance service may have to come from the community nursing budget. There is an additional concern that because of the cost, purchasers may consider the use of a three-layer compression bandage, the effectiveness of which is still being researched. This case study raises questions of how to sustain research-based practice developments in an age of limited resources and health care rationing. We would argue that the responsibility does not rest with individual practitioners alone, but must be placed within the context of organisations and their policies, with due consideration being accorded to the ethical management of care and the involvement of, and dialogue with, informed members of the local community.

SOME IDEAS FOR A NEW MODEL FOR ASSESSING FACTORS FOR IMPLEMENTING RESEARCH

Listening and being able to hear what those around us – colleagues and patients – have to say is a common thread weaving its way through all of the case studies contained in this chapter. This is a central tenet of participatory research, which aims to enable those whose voices have no outlet to pose the problems and questions they feel to be in need of exploration, and to involve them, in a meaningful way, in achieving beneficial change, the success of which they can share in (cf. Chapter 8 for a discussion of critical theory and feminism). To implement research in a fashion that is truly participative requires structures and mechanisms that promote communication and collaboration, ideally across disciplines. Building relationships that facilitate participative inquiry and research-based practice development takes time and involves establishing trust and responding to the concerns expressed by those involved in a genuine and sensitive manner. Strong feelings are often evoked when change is mooted, and this needs recognition.

Health care professionals who achieve change and develop practice are often possessed of a vision that they will readily share given the opportunity. Talking to nurses who had successfully led change, we were struck by the passionate ways in which they expressed their motivations. One nurse spoke of the 'sea of human suffering' in relation to people living with leg ulcers; another of her concern with regard to effecting change in the documentation and practice of nursing care that 'no-one understands how difficult it is to do the job of a nurse'; whilst a third felt it to be imperative that we question our right to assume that we know what it is that patients want. It was also evident that leaders of change had taken time to enable nurses to voice their concerns, to encourage some consensus about the focus of the work, and to promote ownership of it.

There is no doubt that seniority in the nursing hierarchy matters when it comes to disseminating and implementing research. Having power to negotiate is not something that is widely commented upon when it comes to assessing influential factors, yet it is crucial. As one contributor told us, in order to get certain staff to respond to her letters, she needed to go through the Director of Nursing Services. The National Health Service is a class-bound structure characterised by hierarchies that are highly bureaucratic and impersonal, and these can impede creativity and flexibility. Few mechanisms exist to challenge these structures, and the process of bringing about change usually requires the stamp of authority, or as one nurse put it, 'a powerful backer who listens' (see also Chapter 8 for a discussion of power). However, it does seem that creating a culture that encourages partnership between, and the participation of, people at different levels in this hierarchy can be achieved by respect for one another and agreement about the aims and purpose of the proposed project. Investment in disseminating and implementing research will only be seen as worthwhile if it is recognised as something worth doing, if it is understood, believed in and valued. The view long held in medicine that science takes precedence above all is a challenge for interdisciplinary working. Doctors often seem to speak a different language from that of nurses, regarding research into such overarching issues as care, beliefs and rights as generating 'soft' (for which read less valid) rather than 'hard' data. This is a cultural as well as a language barrier that has considerable implications when particular kinds of knowledge and ways of producing it and certain soothsayers are valued above others. As Skeggs (1997 p 29) has said, what constitutes knowledge and evidence is constantly changing and is dependent upon our '...positionings and... access...to different ways of knowing and speaking'. It is important to consider our varying positions and perspectives, to reflect on the different meanings that things hold for us, and to scrutinise the investments we have in them, before we act.

If we were to use another, less well-accepted meaning for the word 'scientific', that of being 'assisted by expert knowledge' (Oxford Modern English Dictionary 1994), then we could ground our examination of what is scientific about nursing practice in a thorough investigation of the expert knowledge held by health care professionals in a variety of settings. We might also concede that our patients are repositories of expert knowledge worthy of exploring as well, and consider how ownership of research by service users may increase utilisation of the findings. Separating science and experience would no longer be necessary. In this way we could avoid becoming tyrannised by evidence (Sackett et al 1996) as it is presently constructed as wholly external and untouched by our relationships with one another. Critical reviews of the literature can provide us with the best external evidence for implementing in practice, but they do not offer us absolutes and should not be applied indiscriminately. They require integrating with other forms of evidence derived from the power of human relationships. One community nurse who took part in the EECN Project expressed this as the need to establish what a client knows, and his or her perception of the issues, and to address the feelings involved in the context of his or her relationships with others. She said:

It's a conscious strategy not to have a definitive answer. I can't just tell clients there's no one right answer, just a recognition of the need to work in partnership and enable them to learn and develop in their relationships and to empower them.

Further study of the mechanisms that nurses use to draw upon a matrix of evidence to enhance patient care would benefit those trying to implement research. We need a better understanding of the relationship between evidence and research and the value systems that influence nurses through the decision-making process. In addition, a review is needed of the state of nursing knowledge concerning processual issues, such as the ways in which relationships are built with individuals and communities, and what is often called nursing 'know-how' (e.g. how nurses provide care and comfort in ways that are meaningful for patients). Such work would be a useful adjunct to the reviews of research into the effectiveness of treatments and therapies being carried out by the Cochrane Collaboration and the NHS Centre for Reviews and Dissemination. The importance of focusing, in terms of both the conduct of research and the conduct of care, on the 'how' of what we do, is that both nursing practice and nursing research are 'processes of action', rather than specific behaviours or acts. Both activities also would benefit from an analysis of the political nature of evidence-based practice and the position of nurses within the organisations that they are part of, with regard to their relative lack of status, power and autonomy. As Kitson et al (1997 p 41) have said, 'We still need a lot of investment to describe properly what it is that we do'. Research findings should not just be implemented without regard to this hidden side of nursing. The fact that nursing is not an exact science has been widely commented upon. It is not a process that is conducted solely on a systematic basis without regard for our patients' and our own feelings. At its best, nursing is dynamic, reflexive, responsive and flexible, able to change its focus and direction to meet the needs of clients which are themselves constantly changing. The '...disparate, disordered complexity of elements that make up the socio-cultural world of nursing practice' have been revealed by Street (1992) in her ethnographic study of nursing. It is not a world that is amenable to strict adherence to policies and protocols which do not allow for 'feeling' evidence or the 'compassionate artistry' (Schon 1992) of the expert nurse. It would seem, then, that more sophisticated measures are needed against which to judge research utilisation. Measures that take into account what Rolfe (1997) has called 'fuzzy logic'. He makes the point that '...people do not process information in the linear "if-then" chains of reasoning employed by digital computers'. We might also question our continued struggle to prove that what we do is scientific.

There have always been elements of myth and magic in nursing, and these can be found in research and indeed in medicine as well (May 1994). Facts become yesterday's myths, and yesterday's myths become today's facts upon which practice is based. For example, witness our horror at the use of leeches for blood letting and at leaving maggots to infest a wound. Today these practices are experiencing a revival, and have been trans-formed from myth (a widely held but false notion) into a scientific fact (Godfrey 1997).

A nursing research strategy, dedicated time, and specific posts are all fac-tors that will facilitate dissemination and implementation. Ownership of the project by practitioners is also important. They will need time to reflect on the change proposed and a supportive educational environment in which to do so. It is seldom formally recognised that nurses have differen-tial access to forms of knowledge such as information technology, libraries, books and conferences, and to the capital needed to invest in these sources of knowledge. For example, certain models for promoting change in clini-cal practice appear to be predicated upon classist, and one could argue, racist, assumptions. The 'personal characteristics' of Stocking's (1992) 'lag-gards' who resist change include low social status, low income and older age. The 'innovators' by contrast have high social status, are wealthy, young and well educated, and attend national and international meetings!

This model for promoting change does not acknowledge issues of access and equity of opportunity, or the dangers of characterising those who have less opportunity as dragging their feet (see Chapter 1 for a description of this model).

The impact of change can be considerable. The process of disseminating and implementing research in today's health care climate will usually take place against a backdrop of change. Constant reorganisations are not uncommon; fear of the market economy and its impact on the viability of care provision and educational programmes is widespread. That the world changes is a key insight in terms of considering appropriate strategies for disseminating and implementing research. Participative approaches to research echo these changes through their constant evolution as they are renegotiated and reinterpreted with participants. Skeggs (1994 p 75), a feminist ethnographer, describes this experience. She writes: 'I did not construct the worlds of the young women [who she was studying]. Their worlds are still there now that I am not. Rather I constructed a discursive representation of it'.

In the guest editorial for *Clinical Effectiveness in Nursing* (entitled 'Science now more than ever'), Closs (1997, p 61) points out that the majority of money available for research through the Department of Health Research and Development programme is allocated to studies focused on clinical and cost effectiveness. Funding bodies, she states, '... have the power to determine which theories are to be adopted/tested by researchers, for political, commercial or other reasons'. Can this be ethically and epistemologically legitimate when surely we should be considering what is of relevance to, and meaningful for, our patients, and not just what is financially or commercially viable? That practice developments save money is likely to be high on the list of purchasers' priorities. Short-term contract research designed to bring about rapid change with the maximum cost benefit does not necessarily contribute to the long-term development of a collaborative, participatory research culture. In terms of the macro, it is important to ask whether the dominant political philosophy is supportive of a participative action based approach to research, or whether it is undermined by this quick-fix consultancy, contract culture, sound bite mentality, and a desire for immediate results. Participative inquiry is potentially in contradiction to these values. This contradiction is particularly apparent in the use of consultancy-style action research which puts issues on the agenda that may prioritise the concerns of managers rather than frontline workers.

The NHS Research and Development strategy is committed to making practice research based and requires strategies for dissemination and implementation to be developed. We would argue that it is important that in the dissemination and implementation process, we expose ourselves to a range of theoretical and methodological options in order to evaluate our findings and their relevance to the practice of nursing and the practice of research. We wish to make it clear that it is our view that nursing does not so much need to develop its own paradigm but instead develop its own perspective and stance. We therefore favour an eclectic approach to nursing research. Similarly, Haase & Myers (1988, p 130) suggest, that rather than challenging one paradigm over another:

A reconciliation of ideas is often attained by emphasising the similarities or commonalities while weighing the impact of true differences. Efforts to integrate paradigms may be enhanced by the same process. Although there is a difference in purpose between qualitative and quantitative approaches, it is helpful, for comparison, to view this difference as one of emphasis.

The emphasis in quantitative approaches is described as 'confirmation of theory by explaining' in contrast to the qualitative paradigm which 'has emphasised discovery and meaning by describing'. Understanding therefore, in Haase & Myers' view, becomes 'the orientating factor in reconciling assumptions' underpinning the two paradigms.

A number of models exist for implementing research which incorporate some of the factors that have contributed to the success of the projects included in this chapter. For example, Kitson et al (1996) suggest that a variety of partnerships and conceptual models need to be established in order to achieve the goal of integrating research into practice and rigorously evaluating it. They point to the interrelationship between inductive and deductive approaches, and consider the strengths and weaknesses of both. Research utilisation is seen as an organisational issue, and not just an individual response. The framework that they propose recognises the need for staff to share skills in research and development initiatives and to develop specific expertise in particular areas. In the USA, the Denver Collaborative Research Network (Keefe et al 1988) has formulated a checklist that is indicative of research readiness within an organisation. It includes such items as:

- adequate facilities and resources
- commitment by the nurse administrator
- faculty and student participation
- trained and interested personnel
- meetings to share research articles at local sites.

Here in the UK, the Foundation of Nursing Studies (1996) has identified a number of factors contributing to the establishment of both national and local research implementation cultures. These include:

- the need to consider interprofessional relationships and perceived medical domination in establishing multidisciplinary working
- the development of local research and development strategies; specific research appointments; funding for courses
- research fora such as nursing development units and research units

- proactive research and ethics committees
- greater uptake of continuing education and better links with education providers.

With regard to collaboration between education and practice, French (1996) proposes using a network of 'link practitioners' alongside the identification of sources of information of clinical effectiveness using such resources as the NHS Centre for Reviews and Dissemination and the Cochrane databases.

Returning to the USA, Tornquist et al (1995) find the Stetler & Marram Model for Application of Research Findings to Practice (Stetler 1994) to be useful. Evaluation of research is accompanied by an assessment, involving nurses, of the appropriateness of research-based change in the practice setting. However, the authors are critical of this and other models which do not address the gulf between researchers and clinicians. They allude to the perception of researchers as 'the intelligentsia in nursing' who are far removed from the 'vast army of doers'. They point out that the majority of those attending research conferences are other researchers, that researchers are heard only by other researchers and that the utility of their work for practice is largely unevaluated. In order to reverse this trend, they suggest that researchers and clinicians need to be reconnected as equals and that there needs to be a greater emphasis on utility for practice, where research findings are presented 'ready for use' in a clear and readable format.

With regard to the broader context, much of the nursing literature places the responsibility for service provision upon the individual practitioner. Yet the organisation and policy context are major factors in creating the climate for good practice, of which research dissemination and implementation are a component. One model for achieving success in service-based nursing research programmes appears to us to accommodate such factors, whilst including the other issues that have emerged in the process of presenting the results of our interviews with leaders of the project development initiatives described in this chapter. R Snyder-Halpern (unpublished work, 1991) highlights the importance of:

- compatibility of mission between the organisation and the research being undertaken
- the abilities of the researcher/change agent
- the need for financial support
- access to support services (such as researchers, databases, statisticians, secretarial assistance)
- the power of the change agents
- the work being carried out by change agents/researchers being their prime responsibility.

Reviewed in the light of other models, this is a useful framework which incorporates the organisational aspects that are identified as influential in the successful implementation of research in practice.

However, this should not devalue the personal dimension of visionary leadership and teamwork which contributes to a dynamic research environment. This is evident in the case studies presented here, which have demonstrated amongst participants the development of self-confidence, feelings of empowerment, the reinforcement of the central ethic of care and the desire to make a difference in people's lives.

ACKNOWLEDGEMENTS

The authors would like to thank all those individuals and organisations who described their experiences of practice development for this chapter. We are grateful for both their time and their generosity in sharing these experiences so frankly with us.

REFERENCES

Abel Smith B 1960 A history of the nursing profession. Heinemann, London

Agency for Health Care Policy Research 1995 Patient involvement enhances care for prostate disease. AHCPR News and Notes 187 (September) 11–12

Allen C 1993 Promoting preceptorship. Nursing Times 89(41): 60

Allen D, Benner P, Diekelmann N 1986 Three paradigms for nursing research methodological implications. In: Chinn P (ed) Nursing research methodology. National League for Nursing, New York, pp 23–38

Anglia and Oxford Regional Health Authority 1994 Getting research into practice and purchasing (GRiPP). Four counties approach. NHS Executive Anglia and Oxford, Oxford

Ankney R N, Heilman P, Kolff J 1996 Newspaper coverage of the coronary artery bypass grafting report. Science Communication 18(2): 153–164

Antman E M, Lau J, Kupelnick B, Mosteller F, Chalmers T C 1992 A comparison of results of meta-analyses of randomised controlled trials and recommendations of clinical experts. Journal of the American Medical Association 268: 240–248

Appelby J, Walshe K, Ham C 1995 Acting on the evidence. National Association of Health Authorities and Trusts, Birmingham

Armitage S 1990 Research utilisation in practice. Nurse Education Today 10: 10–15

Atkinson P 1990 The ethnographic imagination. Routledge, London

Avis M, Robinson J 1996 Continuing dilemma in health care research. NT Research 1(1): 9–11

Avorn J, Soumerai S B 1983 Improving drug-therapy decisions through educational outreach. A randomised trial of academic based detailing. New England Journal of Medicine 308: 1457–1466

Baessler C A, Blumberg M, Cunningham J S et al 1994 Medical-surgical nurses utilisation of research methods and products. Medsurg Nursing 3(2): 113–141

Baker D 1983 Care in the geriatric ward: an account of two styles of nurses. In: Wilson-Barnett J (ed) Nursing research: 10 studies in patient care. John Wiley, Chichester

Barnard K 1986 Research utilisation: the clinician's role. Maternal Child Nursing 11(3): 224

Barnard K, Hoehn R E 1978 Nursing child assessment satellite training. In: Duncan R A (ed) Biomedical communications experiments: using the communications technology satellite. Symposium proceedings. US Public Health Service, Department of Health, Education and Welfare, pp 9–27

Barriball K L, While A E, Norman I J 1992 Continuing professional education for qualified nurses: a review of the literature. Journal of Advanced Nursing 17: 1129–1140

Bassett C C 1993 Role of the nurse teacher as researcher. British Journal of Nursing 2(8): 911–918

Bassett C C 1994 Nurse teachers' attitudes to research: a phenomenological study. Journal of Advanced Nursing 19: 585–592

Bayley E W 1988 A meta-analysis of evaluations of the effect of continuing education on clinical practice in the health professions. PhD thesis, University of Pennsylvania

Becher T 1989 Academic tribes and territories: intellectual enquiry and the culture of disciplines. Society for Research into Higher Education, Open University, Buckingham

Beckhard R, Harris R T 1987 Organisational transitions: managing complex change. Addison Wesley, Massachusetts

Benner P 1984 From novice to expert: excellence and power in clinical nursing practice. Addison Wesley, Menlo Park

Benton D 1997 Making choices: the power of information. Nursing Management 3(8): 10–11

Bircumshaw D 1990 The utilisation of research findings in practice. Journal of Advanced Nursing 15: 1272–1280

Blaxter M 1995 Consumers and research in the NHS. Department of Health NHS Executive, Leeds

Bluff R, Holloway I 1994 'They know best'. Womens' perceptions of midwifery care during labour and childbirth. Midwifery 10: 157–164

Blythe J, Royle J A 1993 Assessing nurses' information needs in the work environment. Bulletin of the Medical Librarians Association 81: 433–435

Booth A 1996 Netting the evidence: a SCHARR introduction to evidence based practice on the Internet. Sheffield Centre for Health and Related Research, University of Sheffield

Boothe P 1981 A study to determine the attitude of professional nurses to nursing research. Unpublished doctoral thesis, University of Alabama

Bostrom A C, Malnight M, MacDougall J, Hargis D 1989 Staff nurses' attitudes toward nursing research: a descriptive survey. Journal of Advanced Nursing 14: 915–922

Bostrom J, Suter W N 1993 Research utilisation: making the link to practice. Journal of Nursing Staff Development 9: 28–34

Bostrom J, Wise L 1994 Closing the gap between research and practice. 'Retrieval and Application of Research in Nursing'. Journal of Nursing Administration 24(5): 22–27

Boyce M E 1996 Solidarity and praxis: being a change agent in a university setting. Journal of Organisational Change 8: 58–66

Brasler M E 1993 Predictors of clinical performance of new graduate nurses participating in preceptor orientation programs. Journal of Continuing Education 24(4): 158–165

Braybrooke D, Lindblom C E 1963 A strategy of decision. Free Press, New York

Brazier H, Begley C M 1996 Selecting a database for literature reviews in nursing: MEDLINE or CINAHL? Journal of Advanced Nursing 24: 868–875

Briggs A 1972 Report of the Committee on Nursing, Cmnd 5115. HMSO, London

Brooker C, Collins K, Akehurst R 1996 Coordinated initiative on the research workforce capacity in health and social care. Review activity 2. Sheffield Centre for Health and Related Research, University of Sheffield

Brown J S, Tanner C A, Padrick K P 1984 Nursing's search for scientific knowledge. Nursing Research 33(1): 26–32

Burls A 1997 An evaluation of the impact of half-day workshops teaching critical appraisal skills. Critical Appraisal Skills Project, Anglia and Oxford Region

Butler P W M 1986 Hospital embedding-diffusion mechanisms and nurses' knowledge of an innovation. Unpublished PhD thesis, University of Michigan, Ann Arbor

Butts P A 1982 Dissemination of nursing research findings. Image: Journal of Nursing Scholarship 16(2): 62–64

Caine C, Kenrick M 1997 The role of clinical directorate managers in facilitating evidence-based practice: a report of an exploratory study. Journal of Nursing Management 5: 157–165

Campanario J M 1995 Commentary on influential books and journal articles initially rejected because of negative referees' evaluations. Science Communications 16(3): 304–325

Carper B 1978 Fundamental patterns of knowing in nursing. Journal of Nursing Scholarship 23(3): 13–23

Carr W, Kemmis S 1986 Becoming critical: education knowledge and action research. Falmer Press, London

Carter D 1996 Barriers to the implementation of research findings in practice. Nurse Researcher 4(2): 30–40

Castledine G 1994 Future standards for teaching in nursing. British Journal of Nursing 3(6): 297–298

Cavanagh S, Coffin D 1993 Teaching nursing research. Senior Nurse 13(4): 51–54

Cavanagh S J, Tross G 1996 Utilising research findings in nursing: policy and practice considerations. Journal of Advanced Nursing 24: 1083–1088

Centre for Policy in Nursing Research 1997 Annual report 1996/7. London School of Hygiene and Tropical Medicine, London

Challen V, Kaminski S, Harris P 1996 Research-mindedness in the radiography profession. Radiography 2: 139–151

Chalmers I, Altman D G 1995 Systematic reviews. BMJ Publishing, London

Champion V L, Leach A 1989 Variables related to research utilisation in nursing: an empirical investigation. Journal of Advanced Nursing 14: 705–710

Chandler J 1991 Reforming nurse education I – the reorganisation of nursing knowledge. Nurse Education Today 11: 83-88

Chapman H 1996 Why do nurses not make use of a solid research base? Nursing Times 92(3): 38–39

Cheater F M, Closs S J 1997 The effectiveness of methods of dissemination of clinical guidelines for nursing practice: a selective review. Clinical Effectiveness in Nursing 1: 4–15

Chenitz W C, Sater B, Giefer K 1986 Nurse attitudes towards research and the clinical setting as a research environment. Proceedings of the National Symposium of Nursing Research, Stanford University Press, Palo Alto

Chrane J 1985a Using research in practice. Research utilisation – theoretical perspectives. Western Journal of Nursing Research 7: 261–268

Chrane J 1985b Using research in practice. Research utilisation – nursing models. Western Journal of Nursing Research 7: 494–497

Clark E J, Sleep J 1991 The what and how of teaching research. Nurse Education Today 11: 172–178

Clarke H F, Derrick L, Eivemark J et al 1994 Nurses' experiences with the implementation of a PCA approach: an interagency collaborative study. Registered Nurses Association of British Columbia, Vancouver

Clifford C, Gough S 1990 Nursing research – a skills based introduction. Prentice Hall, London

Clifford C 1993 The role of the nurse teachers in the empowerment of nurses through research. Nurse Education Today 13: 37–54

Closs S J, Cheater F M 1994 Utilisation of nursing research: culture, interest and support. Journal of Advanced Nursing 19: 762–773

Closs S J 1997 Science now more than ever. Clinical Effectiveness in Nursing 1(2): 61–63

Cochrane A L 1972 Effectiveness and efficiency: random reflections on health services. The Rock Carling Fellowship. Cambridge University Press, Cambridge

Coleman J S, Katz E, Menzel H 1966 Medical innovation: a diffusion study. Bobbs-Merrill, Indianapolis

Collins E G 1992 Increasing practice-based research: doctorally prepared clinical nurse specialists may be the answer. Clinical Nurse Specialist 6(2): 196–200

Cooke H 1993 Boundary work in the nursing curriculum: the case of sociology. Journal of Advanced Nursing 18: 1990–1998

Corcoran-Perry S, Graves J 1990 Supplemental information-seeking behaviour of cardiovascular nurses. Research in Nursing and Health 13: 119–127

Cotter A, Smith P 1998 Epilogue: setting new research agendas. In: Smith P (ed) Nursing research: setting new agendas. Arnold, London

Craik C 1997 Research: moving from debate to action. British Journal of Occupational Therapy 60(2): 65–66

Cresswell J 1997 Delivering satisfaction. Nursing Times 93(19): 23–25

Cullum N 1996 Evidence-based nursing: an introduction. Evidence-Based Nursing. Pilot issue: iv–v

Cullum N 1997 Identification and analysis of randomised controlled trials in nursing: a preliminary study. Quality in Health Care 6: 2–6

Culyer A (1994) Supporting research and development in the NHS. HMSO, London

Conduct and Utilisation of Research in Nursing (CURN) Project 1983 Using research to improve nursing practice. Michigan Nurses' Association. Grune & Stratton, Michigan

Dale A E 1994 The theory–theory gap: the challenge for nurse teachers. Journal of Advanced Nursing 20: 521–524

Davidson D, Rhodes D 1996 The virtual university. Nursing Standard 10(27): 21–22

Davies D A, Thomson M, Oxman A D, Haynes R B 1995 Changing physician performance. A systematic review of the effect of continuing medical education strategies. Journal of the American Medical Association 274: 700–705

Davies K 1990 Women, time and the weavings of the strands of everyday life. Avebury, Aldershot

Dawson S 1995 Never mind the solutions: what are the issues? Lesson of industrial technology transfer for quality in health care. Quality in Health Care 4: 197–203

Denzin N 1989 Strategies of multiple triangulation. In: The research act: a theoretical introduction to sociological methods. McGraw Hill, New York, pp 234–247

Department of Health 1989a Priorities in medical research. HMSO, London

Department of Health 1989b Working for patients. HMSO, London

Department of Health 1991 Research for health: a research and development strategy for the NHS. HMSO, London

Department of Health 1992 The health of the nation. A strategy for health in England and Wales. HMSO, London

Department of Health 1993a Research for health. HMSO, London

Department of Health 1993b Report of the task force on the strategy for research in nursing, midwifery and health visiting. HMSO, London

Department of Health 1993c A vision for the future. The nursing, midwifery and health visiting contribution to health and health care. Department of Health, London

Department of Health 1994a Supporting research and development in the NHS. A report for the minister for health by a research and development taskforce chaired by Professor Anthony Culyer. HMSO, London

Department of Health 1994b Testing the vision. NHS Executive, Leeds

Department of Health 1994c Research and development in occupational therapy, physiotherapy and speech and language therapy: a position statement. Department of Health, London

Department of Health 1995a Methods to promote the implementation of research findings in the NHS – priorities for evaluation. Department of Health, Leeds

Department of Health 1995b Consumers and research in the NHS. An R&D contribution to consumer involvement in the NHS. Department of Health, Leeds

Department of Health 1996a Promoting clinical effectiveness: a framework for action in and through the NHS. NHS Executive, Leeds

Department of Health 1996b Research and development: towards an evidence-based health service. Department of Health, London

Department of Health 1996c The National Health Service: a service with ambitions. Stationery Office, London

Department of Health 1997 The new NHS: Modern. Dependable. Stationery Office, London

Dickinson E 1995 Using marketing principles for healthcare development. Quality in Health Care 4: 40–44

Dickson R, Cullum N 1996 Systematic reviews: how to use the information. Nursing Standard 10(20): 32

Dingwall R, McIntosh J 1978 Readings in the sociology of nursing. Churchill Livingstone, Edinburgh

Donald A 1996 Front-line evidence based medicine. NHSE North Thames R & D News, issue 9 (Autumn/Winter)

Dopson S, Mant J, Hicks N 1994 Getting research into practice: facing the issues. Journal of Management in Medicine 8(6): 4–12

Dowie J 1996 'Evidence-based', 'cost-effective' and 'preference-driven' medicine: decision analysis based medical decision making is the prerequisite. Journal of Health Services Research Policy 1(2): 104–113

Dowie J, Elstein A 1988 Professional judgment: a reader in clinical decision making. Cambridge University Press, Cambridge

Droogan J, Sanderson J 1995 An initial survey of practice and service developments within the health care professions in the United Kingdom. NHS Centre for Reviews and Dissemination, York

Droogan J, Cullum N 1998 Systematic reviews in nursing. International Journal of Nursing Studies 35: 13–22

Duffy M 1986 Nursing research at the baccalaureate level. Nursing and Health Care 7(6): 293–295

Dunning M, Cooper S 1996 Setting the PACE. Health Director, June

Easen P, Wilcockson J 1996 Intuition and rational decision making in professional thinking: a false dichotomy? Journal of Advanced Nursing 24: 667–673

Eckerling S, Bergman R, Bar-Tal Y 1988 Perceptions and attitudes of academic nursing students to research. Journal of Advanced Nursing 13: 759–767

Effective Health Care 1994 Implementing clinical practice guidelines: can guidelines be used to improve clinical practice? Bulletin no. 8, Nuffield Institute for Health, University of Leeds & NHS CRD, University of York

Ehrenfeld M, Eckerling S 1991 Perceptions and attitudes of registered nurses: a comparison with a previous study. Journal of Advanced Nursing 16: 224–232

Ellis J, Mulligan I, Rowe J, Sackett D L 1995 Inpatient general medicine is evidence-based. A-Team Nuffield Department of Clinical Medicine. Lancet 345: 407–410

Elwood J M 1988 Causal relationships in medicine: a practical system for critical appraisal. Oxford Medical Publications, Oxford

Emery D 1996 Education for nurses and midwives at a distance. Health Informatics 2: 40–43

English I 1994 Nursing as a research-based profession: 22 years after Briggs. British Journal of Nursing 3(8): 402–406

English National Board for Nursing, Midwifery and Health Visiting 1990 Framework for continuing professional education for nurses, midwives and health visitors. Summary report for educationalists. Project paper three. ENB, London

English National Board for Nursing, Midwifery and Health Visiting 1995 National consultation to identify research priorities in nursing, midwifery and health visiting education and practice. Report of the Consultation and Outcomes. ENB, London

Entwistle V, Watt I S, Herring J E 1996 Information about health care effectiveness. Kings Fund, London

Evans C E, Haynes R B, Birkett N J 1986 Does a mailed continuing education program improve physician performance? Results of a randomised trial in antihypertensive care. Journal of the American Medical Association 255: 501–504

Eve R 1995 Implementing clinical change: learning from the US experience. FACTS programme. Sheffield Centre for Health and Related Research, University of Sheffield.

Ferguson K E, Jinks A M 1994 Integrating what is taught with what is practised in the nursing curriculum: a multi-dimensional model. Journal of Advanced Nursing 20: 687–695

Firlit S, Walsh M, Kemp M 1987 Nursing research in practice: a survey of research utilisation content in master's degree programs. Western Journal of Nursing Research 9: 612–616

Fisher R F, Strank R A 1971 An investigation into the reading habits of qualified nurses. Nursing Times 67: 245–247

Floyd J A 1996 An undergraduate research course: emphasis on research utilisation. Journal of Nursing Education 35(4): 185–187

Foot P 1974 Theories of ethics. Open University Press, Milton Keynes

Ford P, Walsh M 1994 New rituals for old. Nursing through the looking glass. Butterworth-Heinemann, Oxford

Foucault M 1976 The birth of the clinic. Tavistock, London

Foucault M 1980 Michel Foucault: power/knowledge: selected interviews and other writings, 1972–1977. Harvester Press, Brighton

Foundation of Nursing Studies 1996 Reflection for action. Foundation of Nursing Studies, London

Francke A L, Garssen B, Huijer Abu-Saad H 1995 Determinants of change in nurses' behaviour after continuing education: a literature review. Journal of Advanced Nursing 21: 371–377

Freemantle N, Watt I 1994 Dissemination: implementing the findings of research. Health Libraries Review 11: 133–137

Freemantle N, Harvey E L, Grimshaw J M et al 1996 The effectiveness of printed educational materials in improving the behaviour of health care professionals and patient outcomes. In: Bero L, Grilli R, Grimshaw J, Oxman A (eds) Collaboration on effective professional practice module of the Cochrane database of systematic reviews. Cochrane Library, Oxford

French B 1996 Networking for research dissemination: collaboration between education and practice. NT Research 1(2): 113–118

Fretwell J E 1982 Ward teaching and learning. Royal College of Nursing, London

Friere P 1985 The politics of education: culture, power and liberation (Macedo D, transl). Bergey & Garvin, Westport Connecticut

Friere P 1994 Pedagogy of the oppressed, 20th edn. Continuum, New York

Funk S G, Tornquist E M, Champagne M T 1989 A model for improving dissemination of nursing research. Western Journal of Nursing Research 11: 361–367

Funk S, Champagne M T, Wiese R, Tornquist E M 1991 BARRIERS: the barriers to research utilisation scale. Applied Nursing Research 4: 39–45

Gadamer H G 1976 Philosophical hermeneutics (Linge D E transl). University of California Press, Berkeley

Gibbons L L, Nowonty H, Schwartzmann S P, Scott P, Trow P 1994 The new production of knowledge: the dynamics of science and research in contemporary societies. Sage, London

Gill P, Dowell A C, Neal R D, Smith N, Heywood P, Wilson A F 1996 Evidence-based general practice: a retrospective study of interventions in one training practice. British Medical Journal 312: 812–821

Glasser E M, Abelson H H, Garrison K N 1983 Putting knowledge to use: facilitating the diffusion of knowledge and the implementation of planned change. Jossey-Bass, San Francisco

Godfrey K 1997 Use of leeches and leech saliva in clinical practice. Nursing Times 93(9): 62–63

Goode C J, Bulechek G M 1992 Research utilisation: an organisational process that enhances quality of care. Journal of Nursing Care and Quality (special report): 27–35

Goode C J, Lovett M K, Hayes J E et al 1987 Use of research based knowledge in clinical practice. Journal of Nursing Administration 17: 11–18

Gordon C 1995 Health telematics for clinical guidelines and protocols. In: Laires M F, Ladeira M J, Christensen J P (eds) Health in the new communications age. IOS Press, Amsterdam, pp 274–278

Gould D 1986 Pressure sore prevention and treatment: an example of nurses' failure to implement research findings. Journal of Advanced Nursing 11: 389–394

Graves J R 1990 A research-knowledge system (ARKS) for storing, managing and modelling knowledge from the scientific literature. Advances in Nursing Science 13(2): 34–45

Greenfield S, Kaplan S, Ware J E 1985 Expanding patient involvement in care: effects on patient outcomes. Annals of Internal Medicine 102: 520–528

Greenhalgh T 1996 Is my practice evidence-based? British Medical Journal 313: 957–958

Greer A L 1988 The state of the art versus the state of the science: the diffusion of new medical technologies into practice. International Journal of Technology Assessment in Health Care 4: 5–26

Griffiths J, Luker K 1997 A barrier to clinical effectiveness: the etiquette of district nursing. Clinical Effectiveness in Nursing 1(30): 121–130

Gunn L 1989 A public management approach to the NHS. Health Services Management Research 2: 10–19

Haase J E, Meyers S T 1988 Reconciling paradigm assumptions of qualitative and quantitative research. Western Journal of Nursing Research 10: 128–137

Habermas J 1970 Knowledge and human interest (Shapiro J transl). Heinemann, London

Hagell 1989 Nursing knowledge: women's knowledges. A sociological perspective. Journal of Advanced Nursing 14: 226–233

Haig P 1993 Nursing journals: are nurses using them? Nursing Standard 8(1): 22–25

Haines A, Jones R 1994 Implementing findings of research. British Medical Journal 308: 1488–1492

Hall J M, Stevens P E 1991 Rigour in feminist research. Advances in Nursing Science 13(3): 16–29

Halpert H P 1966 Communication as a basic tool in practical uses of research findings. Community Mental Health Journal 2(3): 231–236

Hardey M 1994 The dissemination and utilisation of research. In: Hardey M, Mulhall A (eds) Nursing research: theory and practice. Chapman & Hall, London, pp 163–185

Harris M 1992 The impact of research findings on current practice in relieving postpartum perineal pain in a large district general hospital. Midwifery 8: 125–131

Harrison LL, Lowery B, Bailey P 1991 Changes in nursing students' knowledge about and attitudes towards research following an undergraduate research course. Journal of Advanced Nursing 16: 807–812

Hart C, Lekander B, Bartels D, Tebbin B 1987 Clinical nurse specialist: an institutional process for establishing priorities. Journal of Nursing Administration 17: 31

Hathaway D 1986 Effects of preoperative instruction on post-operative outcomes: a meta analysis. Nursing Research 35: 269–275

Havelock R G 1969 Planning for innovation through dissemination and utilisation of scientific knowledge. Centre for Research on Utilisation of Scientific Knowledge, Institute for Social Research, University of Michigan, Ann Arbor

Havelock R G, Havelock M 1973 Training for change agents. Centre for Research on Utilisation of Scientific Knowledge, Institute for Social Research, University of Michigan, Ann Arbor

Healy 1997 Architects of the great depression. The Times Higher Educational Supplement 30 May: 16

Hefferin E A, Horsley J A, Ventura M R 1982 Promoting research based nursing: the nurse administrator's role. Journal of Nursing Administration 12: 34–41

Hendry J 1997 The Cumbria genesis project (Millenium Project no MC/N/1809). Cumbria Lifelong Education Project, Cumbria County Council, Carlisle

Henry S B 1995 Nursing informatics: state of the science. Journal of Advanced Nursing 22: 1182–1192

Hickey M 1990 The role of the clinical nurse specialist in the research utilisation process. Clinical Nurse Specialist 4(2): 93–96

Hicks C 1992 Research in midwifery: are midwives their own worst enemies? Midwifery 8: 12–18

Hicks C 1993 A survey of midwives' attitudes to, and involvement in, research: the first stage in identifying needs for a staff development programme. Midwifery 9: 51–62

Hicks C 1994 Bridging the gap between research and practice: an assessment of the value of a study day in developing critical research reading skills in midwives. Midwifery 10: 18–25

Hicks C 1995 The shortfall in published research: a study of nurses' research and publication activities. Journal of Advanced Nursing 21: 594–604

Hicks C 1996 A study of nurses' attitudes towards research: a factor analytic approach. Journal of Advanced Nursing 23: 373–379

Hicks C, Hennessy D 1997 Mixed messages in nursing research: their contribution to the persisting hiatus between evidence and practice. Journal of Advanced Nursing 25: 595–601

Hicks C, Hennessy D, Cooper J, Barwell F 1996 Investigating attitudes to research in primary health care teams. Journal of Advanced Nursing 24: 1033–1041

Hockey L 1985 Nursing research, mistakes and misconceptions. Churchill Livingstone, Edinburgh

Holland C K 1993 An ethnographic study of nursing culture as an explanation for determining the existence of a system of ritual. Journal of Advanced Nursing 18: 1461–1470

Holter I M, Schwartz-Barcott D 1993 Action research: what is it? How has it been used and how can it be used in nursing? Journal of Advanced Nursing 18: 298–304

Hope T 1996 Evidence-based patient choice. Kings Fund, London

Horsley J A, Chrane J, Crabtree M K 1983 Using research to improve nursing practice. A guide. Grune & Stratton, New York

House of Lords' Select Committee on Science and Technology 1988 Priorities in medical research. 3rd report: 1987–88 session. HMSO, London

Huber G L 1994 Clinical nurse specialist and staff nurse colleagues in integrating nursing research with clinical practice. Clinical Nurse Specialist 8(1): 118–121

Huber M L 1981 The effects of preceptorship and internship orientation programs on graduate nurse performance. Unpublished PhD thesis, Wayne State University, Michigan

Huberman M 1987 Steps toward an integrated model of research utilisation. Knowledge: Creation, Diffusion, Utilization 8(4): 586–611

Hunt J 1981 Indications for nursing practice: the use of research findings. Journal of Advanced Nursing 6: 189–194

Hunt J 1984 Why don't we use these findings? Nursing Mirror 158(8): 29

Hunt J M 1996 Barriers to research utilisation. Journal of Advanced Nursing 23: 423–425

Hunt J 1997 Towards evidence based practice. Nursing Management 4: 14–17

Hunt M 1987 The process of translating research findings into nursing practice. Journal of Advanced Nursing 12: 101–110

Hunt V, Stark J L, Fisher F, Hegedus K, Joy L, Woldum K 1983 Networking: a managerial strategy for research development in a service setting. Journal of Nursing Administration 13(7/8): 27–33

Itano J K, Warren J, Ishida D N 1987 A comparison of role conceptions and role deprivation of baccalaureate students in nursing participating in a preceptorship or a traditional clinical program. Journal of Nursing Education 26: 69–73

Jacobsen B S, Meininger J C 1985 The designs and methods of published nursing research. Nursing Research 34: 306–312

Jacoby I, Clark S 1986 Direct mailing as a means of dissemination NIH consensus statements. Journal of the American Medical Association 255: 1328–1330

Jenkins D 1991 Investigations: how to get from guidelines to protocols. British Medical Journal 303: 323–324

Jordan S 1994 Should nurses be studying bioscience? A discussion paper. Nurse Education Today 14: 417–426

Jowett S, Walton I, Payne S 1994 Challenges and change in nurse education: a study of the implementation of Project 2000. National Foundation for Educational Research in England and Wales, Slough

Jowett S 1995 Project 2000 in practice – a follow-up study of people from the first intakes of the diploma in nursing course. National Foundation for Educational Research, Slough

Kanouse D E, Jacoby I 1988 When does information change practitioners' behaviour? International Journal of Technology Assessment in Health Care 4: 27–33

Keefe M, Pepper G, Stoner M 1988 Toward research-based nursing practice: the Denver Collaborative Research Network. Applied Nursing Research 1(3): 109

Kendrick K, Simpson A 1992 The nurses' reformation: philosophy and pragmatics of Project 2000. In: Soothill K, Henry C, Kendrick K (eds) Themes and perspectives in nursing. Chapman & Hall, London, pp 91–100

Kilby S A, Fishel C C, Gupta A D 1989 Access to nursing information resources. Image: Journal of Nursing Scholarship 21(1): 26–30

Kilby S A, Rupp L F, Fishel C C, Brecht M 1991 Changes in nursing's periodical literature 1975–1985. Nursing Outlook 39(2): 82–86

Kirchoff K T, Beck S L 1995 Using the journal club as a component of the research utilisation process. Heart and Lung 24(3): 246–250

Kirk S 1996 The NHS research and development strategy. In: Baker M, Kirk S (eds) Research and development for the NHS: evidence, evaluation and effectiveness. Radcliffe Medical Press, Oxford

Kirk S, Carlisle C, Luker K A 1996 The changing academic role of the nurse teacher in the United Kingdom. Journal of Advanced Nursing 24: 1054–1062

Kitson A, Ahmed L B, Harvey G, Seers K, Thompson D R 1996 From research to practice: one organisational model for promoting research-based practice. Journal of Advanced Nursing 23: 430–440

Kitson A, McMahon A, Rafferty A M, Scott E 1997 On developing an agenda to influence policy in health-care research for effective nursing: a description of a national R&D priority setting exercise. NT Research 2(5): 323–334

Knott J, Wildavasky A 1980 If dissemination is the solution, what is the problem? Knowledge: Creation, Diffusion, Utilization 1(4): 537–578

Kramer M 1974 Reality shock: why nurses leave nursing. Mosby, St Louis

Kramer M, Holaday B, Hoeffer B 1981 The teaching of nursing research – part ii. A literature review of teaching strategies. Nurse Educator 6(2): 30–35

Kreuger J C, Nelson A H, Wolanin M O 1978 Nursing research: development, collaboration, and utilisation. Aspen Systems, Germantown

Kuhn T 1970 The structure of scientific revolutions, 2nd edn. University of Chicago Press, Chicago

Lacey E A 1994 Research utilisation in practice – a pilot study. Journal of Advanced Nursing 19: 987–995

Lacey E A 1996 Facilitating research-based practice by educational intervention. Nurse Education Today 16: 296–301

La Monica E 1994 Management in health. A theoretical and experiential approach. Macmillan, Basingstoke

LaPorte R E 1994 Global public health and the information superhighway. British Medical Journal 308(6945): 1651–1652

LaPorte R E, Marler S, Akazawa F et al 1995 The death of biomedical journals. British Medical Journal 310: 1387–1389

Lathlean J 1987 Are you prepared to be a staff nurse? Nursing Times 83(36): 25–27

Lathlean J 1989 Research and evaluation. In: Dodwell M, Lathlean J (eds) Management and professional development for nurses. Harper & Row, London

Lathlean J, Smith G, Bradley S 1986 Post-registration development schemes. NERU report no. 4. Nursing Research Unit, King's College, University of London, London

Latour B, Woolgar S 1979 Laboratory life: the social construction of scientific facts. Sage, Beverley Hills

Lau J L, Antman E M, Jimenez-Silva J , Kupelnick B, Mosteller F, Chalmers T C 1992 Cumulative meta-analysis of therapeutic trials for myocardial infarction. New England Journal of Medicine 327: 248–254

Lawler J 1991 Behind the screens nursing. Churchill Livingstone, Edinburgh

Lawler J 1997 The body in nursing. Churchill Livingstone, Edinburgh

Lawson N 1996 Is it the end for nurses? The Times 31 December

Le May A, Mulhall A, Alexander C 1997 The research culture – myth or reality from a nursing and management perspective. Proceedings of the RCN Research Society Conference, Newcastle, April

Le May A, Mulhall A, Alexander C 1998 Bridging the research practice gap: exploring the research cultures of practitioners and managers. Journal of Advanced Nursing 28: 428–437

Le Var R, Steadman S 1996 Teaching research in nursing and midwifery curricula. Occasional report. English National Board for Nursing, Midwifery and Health Visiting, London

Lewin K 1946 Action research and minority problems. Journal of Social Issues 2: 34–46

Lewin K 1951 Field theory in the social sciences. Harper, New York

Lindblom C E, Cohen D K 1979 Usable knowledge: social science and social problem solving. Yale University Press, New Haven

Linde B J 1989 The effectiveness of three interventions to increase research utilisation. Unpublished PhD thesis, University of Michigan, Ann Arbor

Lippitt R, Watson J, Westley B 1958 The dynamics of planned change. Harcourt Brace Jovanovich, New York

Little P, Smith L, Cantrell T, Chapman J, Langridge J, Pickering R 1996 General practitioners' management of acute back pain: a survey of reported practice compared with clinical guidelines. British Medical Journal 312: 485–488

Logue R 1996 Is nursing research detrimental to nursing education and practice? Nurse Researcher 4(1): 63–69

Lomas J 1991 Words without action? The production, dissemination and impact of consensus recommendations. Annual Review of Public Health 12: 41–65

Lomas J, Haynes R B 1987 A taxonomy and critical review of tested strategies for the application of clinical practice recommendations: from 'official' to 'individual' clinical policy. American Journal of Preventative Medicine 4: 77–95

Long A 1996 Health services research – a radical approach to cross the research and development divide? In: Baker M, Kirk S (eds) Research and development for the NHS: evidence evaluation and effectiveness. Radcliffe Medical Press, Oxford, pp 51–63

Longman 1991 Dictionary of contemporary English. Longman, Harlow

Lorentzon M 1995 Multidisciplinary collaboration: life line or drowning pool for nurse researchers? Journal of Advanced Nursing 22: 825

Ludeman R 1980 The language and importance of nursing research. Western Journal of Nursing Research 2: 432–434

Luker K A, Kenrick M 1992 An exploratory study of the sources of influence on the clinical decisions of community nurses. Journal of Advanced Nursing 17: 457–466

Luker K A, Kenrick M 1995 Towards knowledge-based practice; an evaluation of a method of dissemination. International Journal of Nursing Studies 32(1): 59–67

Lyte V, Kershaw B 1994 Watch and learn. Nursing Times 90(42): 44–46

Maben J, Macleod Clark J 1996a Making the transition from student to staff nurse. Nursing Times 92(44): 28–31

Maben J, Macleod Clark J 1996b Preceptorship and support for staff: the good and the bad. Nursing Times 92(51): 35–38

McIntosh J 1995 Barriers to research implementation. Nurse Researcher 2(4): 83–87

McKenna H 1995 Dissemination and application of mental health nursing research. British Journal of Nursing 4(21): 1257–1263

Macleod Clark J, Maben J, Jones K 1996 Project 2000: perceptions of the philosophy and practice of nursing. Final report, English National Board for Nursing, Midwifery and Health Visiting, London

MacGuire J M 1990 Putting nursing research findings into practice: research utilisation as an aspect of the management of change. Journal of Advanced Nursing 15: 614–620

McLoughlin C 1996 Purchasing R and D in nursing: its role in the shared agenda to improve the NHS. NT Research 1(6): 409–411

McPhelim J, Sarvesvaran J 1997 Face to face. Lung cancer specialist and respiratory registrar. Nursing Times 93(44): 40–41

Marsh G W, Brown T L 1992 The measurement of nurses' attitudes towards research and the research environment in clinical settings. Journal of Clinical Nursing 1: 315–322

Matthews R 1995 Storming the barricades. New Scientist 17 June

May A K 1994 Abstract knowing: the case for magic in method. In: Morse J M (ed) Issues in qualitative research methods. Sage, London

Mayhew P A 1994 Academic/practice collaboration for nursing research. Medsurg Nursing 3(3): 210, 230–231

Meah S, Luker K A, Cullum N A 1996 An exploration of midwives' attitudes to research and perceived barriers to research utilisation. Midwifery 12: 73–84

Meerabeau L 1995 The nature of practitioner knowledge. In: Reed J, Procter S (eds) Practitioner research in health care. Chapman & Hall, London, pp 32–45

Melia K 1982 'Telling it as it is' – qualitative methodology and nursing research: understanding the student nurse's world. Journal of Advanced Nursing 7: 327–336

Melia K 1987 Learning and working: the occupational socialization of nurses. Tavistock, London

Meyer J 1995 Stages in the process: a personal account. Nurse Researcher 2(3): 24–37

Meyer J, Batehup L 1997 Action research in health care practice: nature, present concerns and future possibilities. NT Research 2(3): 175–184

Miller P 1996 Dissemination and utilisation of research: outcome behaviours at the baccalaureate level. Journal of Nursing Education 35(4): 175–177

Miller J R, Messenger S R 1978 Obstacles to applying nursing research findings. American Journal of Nursing 78: 632–634

Moody L E, Wilson M E, Smyth K, Schwartz R, Tittle M, Van Cott M L 1988 Analysis of a decade of nursing practice research 1977–1986. Nursing Research 37(7): 374–379

Moorbath P 1996 Nursing libraries: a survey of nurses' access to facilities. Nursing Standard 10(18): 44–46

Morris B 1996 News and views – informing children about their illnesses. International Journal of Health Care Quality Assurance 9(3): 1–2

Morse J M, Miles M W, Clark D A, Doberneck B M 1994 'Sensing' patient needs: exploring concepts of nursing insight and receptivity used in nursing assessment. Scholarly Inquiry for Nursing Practice 8(3): 233–253

Mortensen R A, Nielsen G H 1995 TELENURSING. In: Laires M F, Ladeira M J, Christensen J P (eds) Health in the new communications age. IOS Press, Amsterdam

Morton-Cooper A, Palmer A 1993 Mentoring and preceptorship: a guide to support roles in clinical practice. Blackwell Scientific, Oxford

Muir Gray J A 1997 Evidence-Based Healthcare – how to make health policy and management decisions. Churchill Livingstone, Edinburgh

Mulhall A 1995 Nursing research: what difference does it make? Journal of Advanced Nursing 21: 576–583

Mulhall A 1996 Epidemiology, nursing and healthcare – a new perspective. Macmillan, Basingstoke

Mulhall A 1997 Nursing research: our world not theirs? Journal of Advanced Nursing 25: 969–976

Mulhall A, Le May A, Alexander C 1996 The utilisation of research in nursing. A report of a phenomenological study involving nurses and managers. In: Reflection for Action. Foundation of Nursing Studies, London, pp 12–17

Mulrow C 1987 The medical review article: state of the science. Annals of Internal Medicine 106: 485–488

Murphy E, Freston M S 1991 An analysis of theory–research linkages in published gerontological nursing studies: 1983–1989. Advances in Nursing Science 13(4): 1–13

Murray M, Reid N, Robinson G, Sloan J P 1990 Attitudes towards research: report of a survey of the views of nursing service and nursing educational staff in Northern Ireland. Occasional paper no. 1. National Board for Nursing, Midwifery and Health Visiting for Northern Ireland, Belfast

Musson G 1996 Qualitative Evaluation of the FACTS Aspirin Programme – interim report. Sheffield Business School, University of Sheffield

Myco F 1980 Nursing research information: are nurse educators and practitioners seeking it out? Journal of Advanced Nursing 5: 637–646

Myrick F 1988 Preceptorship – is it the answer to the problems in clinical teaching? Journal of Nursing Education 27(3): 136–138

Naylor C D 1995 Grey zones of clinical practice: some limits to evidence-based medicine. Lancet 345: 840–842

Nelson D 1995 Research into research practice. Accident and Emergency Nursing 3: 184–189

Newton CA 1995 Action research: application in practice. Nurse Researcher 2(3): 60–71

NHS Centre for Reviews and Dissemination 1996 Undertaking systematic reviews of research on effectiveness: CRD guidelines for those carrying out or commissioning reviews. CRD report 4. NHS Centre for Reviews and Dissemination, York

NHS Executive 1996. Promoting clinical excellence: a framework for action in and through the NHS. Department of Health, Leeds

NHS Management Enquiry 1983 The Griffiths report. HMSO, London

Nielsen J M 1990 Introduction. In: Nielsen J M (ed) Feminist research methods: exemplary readings in the social sciences. Westview Press, Boulder, Colorado, pp 1–37

Nolan PW 1989 Psychiatric nursing past and present: the nurse's viewpoint. Unpublished PhD thesis, University of Bath

Norris C M 1982 (ed) Concept clarification in nursing. Aspen, Colorado

Orr J G 1987 Why shouldn't we be clever? Nursing Times 83(35): 24

Orton H 1981 Ward learning climate. Royal College of Nursing, London

Overfield T, Duffy M E 1984 Research on teaching research in the baccalaureate nursing curriculum. Journal of Advanced Nursing 9: 189–196

Owen P 1995 Clinical practice and medical research: bridging the divide between the two cultures. British Journal of General Practice 45: 557–560

Oxford Modern English Dictionary 1994. Clarendon Press, Oxford

Oxman A 1994 No magic bullets: a systematic review of 102 trials of interventions to help health care professionals deliver services more effectively or efficiently. Report to North East Thames Regional Health Authority

Pattison S 1996 Change management in the British National Health Service: a worm's eye critique. Health Care Analysis 4: 252–258

Pearcey P A 1995 Achieving research based nursing practice. Journal of Advanced Nursing 22: 33–39

Pearcey P, Draper P 1996 Using the diffusion of innovation model to influence practice: a case study. Journal of Advanced Nursing 23: 714–721

Pembrey S 1982 The ward sister – key to nursing. Royal College of Nursing, London

Perkins E R 1992 Teaching research to nurses: issues for tutor training. Nurse Education Today 12: 252–257

Peters D A 1992 Implementation of research findings. Health Bulletin 50(1): 68–77

Pettigrew A M 1985 The awakening giant: contingency and change in ICI. Blackwell, London

Phillips T, Schostak J, Bedford H, Robinson J E 1993 Assessment of competencies in nursing and midwifery education and training (the Ace project). Research highlights no. 4. English National Board for Nursing, Midwifery and Health Visiting, London

Plant R 1987 Managing change and making it stick. Fontana, London

Pond E F, Bradshaw M J 1996 Attitudes of nursing students towards research: a participatory exercise. Journal of Nursing Education 35(4): 182–185

Pope C, Mays N 1995 Reaching the parts other methods cannot reach: an introduction to qualitative methods in health and health services research. British Journal of Medicine 311: 42–45

Porter S 1993 Nursing research conventions: objectivity or obfuscation? Journal of Advanced Nursing 18: 137–143

Porter S, Ryan S 1996 Breaking the boundaries between nursing and sociology: a critical realist ethnography of the theory–practice gap. Journal of Advanced Nursing 24: 413–420

Rafferty A M, Allcock N, Lathlean J 1996 The theory practice gap: taking issue with the issue. Journal of Advanced Nursing 23: 685–691

Rafferty A M, Traynor M 1997 Quality and quantity in research policy for nursing. NT Research 2(1): 16–27

Ranade W 1994 A future for the NHS? Longman, London

Ratcliffe J W, Gonzalez-del-Ville A 1988 Rigor in health-related research: towards an expanded conceptualisation. International Journal of Health Services 18: 361–392

Rayner C 1997 A Claire view. Nursing Times 93(8): 34–35

Reed J, Robbins L 1991 Research rituals. Nursing Times 87(23): 50–51

Resnik D 1996 Data falsification in clinical trials. Science Communication 18(1): 49–58

Richardson A, Jackson C, Sykes W 1990 Taking research seriously: means of improving and assessing the use and dissemination of research. HMSO, London

Rizzuto C, Bostrom J, Suter W N, Chenitz W C 1994 Predictors of nurses' involvement in research activities. Western Journal of Nursing Research 16: 193–204

Roberts J, While A, Fitzpatrick J 1995 Information-seeking strategies and data utilisation: theory and practice. International Journal of Nursing Studies 32(6): 601–611

Robinson J 1993 Problems with paradigms in a caring profession. In: Kitson A (ed) Nursing: art and science. Chapman & Hall, London, pp 72–84

Robinson J, Rex S, Boorman L 1993 Project 2000 and local staff nurse development. Senior Nurse 13(4): 32–35

Robinson K, Vaughan B (eds) 1992 Knowledge for nursing practice. Butterworth-Heinemann, London

Rodgers S 1994 An exploratory study of research utilisation by nurses in general medical and surgical wards. Journal of Advanced Nursing 20: 904–911

Rogers E M 1983 Diffusion of innovations. Free Press, New York

Rogers E M 1995 Diffusion of innovations, 4th edn. Free Press, New York

Rogers E M, Shoemaker F F 1971 Communication of innovations: a cross cultural approach. Free Press, New York

Rolfe G 1994 Towards a new model of nursing research. Journal of Advanced Nursing 19: 969–975

Rolfe G 1997 Science, abduction and the fuzzy nurse: an exploration of expertise. Journal of Advanced Nursing 25: 1070–1075

Ryan D 1989 Project 1999 – The support hierarchy as the management contribution to Project 2000. Evaluation project discussion paper no. 4. Department of Nursing Studies, University of Edinburgh

Sackett D L 1996 Evidence based medicine. Churchill Livingstone, London

Sackett D L, Haynes R B 1995 On the need for evidence-based medicine. Evidence Based Medicine 1: 5–6

Sackett D L, Haynes R B, Guyatt G H, Tugwell P 1991 Clinical epidemiology: a basic science for clinical medicine. Little Brown, Boston

Sackett D L, Rosenberg W, Haynes R B, Richardson W S 1996 Evidence-based medicine: what it is and what it isn't. British Medical Journal 312: 71–72

Sackett D L, Richardson W S, Rosenberg W, Haynes R B 1997 Evidence based medicine. How to practice and teach EBM. Churchill Livingstone, Edinburgh

Salmon B 1968 Report of the committee on senior nurse staff structure. HMSO, London

Salvage J 1985 The politics of nursing. Butterworth-Heinemann, Oxford

Sarvimaki A 1988 Nursing as a moral, practical, communicative and creative activity. Journal of Advanced Nursing 13: 462–467

Savage J 1995 Nursing intimacy: an ethnographic approach to nurse patient interaction. Scutari Press, London

Schare B L, Dunn S C, Clark H M, Soled S W, Gilman B R 1991 The effects of interactive video on cognitive achievement and attitude toward learning. Journal of Nursing Education 30(3): 109–113

Schon D A 1983 The reflective practitioner. Basic Books, New York

Schon D A 1987 Educating the reflective practitioner. Jossey-Bass, San Francisco

Schon D 1992 The crisis of professional knowledge and the pursuit of an epistemology of practice. Journal of Interprofessional Care 6(1): 49–63

Schulz K, Chalmers I, Hayes R J, Altman D G 1995 Empirical evidence of bias. Dimensions of methodological quality associated with estimates of treatment effects in controlled clinical trials. Journal of the American Medical Association 273: 408–412

Schumacker K Gortner S 1992 (Mis)conceptions and reconceptions about traditional science. Advances in Nursing Science 14(4): 226–232

Science Citation Index 1996 Journal citation reports. Institute for Scientific Information, Uxbridge

Scientific Basis of Health Services Conference, 2–5 October 1995 Queen Elizabeth Conference Centre. Audiotapes available from QED Recording Services, Lancaster Road, New Barnett, Herts EN4 8AS. Tel. 0181 441 7722, Fax 0181 441 0777

Scott A, Campbell H, Gorman D 1994 Preventing SIDS. Evidence of health visitors changing their practice. Health Visitor 67(11): 380–381

Scottish Office Home and Health Department 1991 A strategy for nursing research in Scotland. Chief Area Nursing Officers and the Scottish Office Home and Health Department, Edinburgh

Seccombe I, Smith G 1997 Taking part: registered nurses and the labour market in 1997. A summary. Report 338. Institute for Employment Studies, Brighton

Seers K, Goodman C 1987 Perceptions of pain. Nursing Times 83(48): 37–39

Seligman M E P 1975 Helplessness: on depression, development and death. Freeman, San Francisco

Shand M 1987 Unreasonable expectations? Nursing Times 83(36): 28–30

Sheehan J 1990 Investigating change in a nursing context. Journal of Advanced Nursing 15: 819–824

Sheehan J 1994 A journal club as a teaching and learning strategy in nurse teacher education. Journal of Advanced Nursing 19: 572–576

Shin J H, Haynes R B, Jonson M E 1993 Effect of problem-based, self-directed undergraduate education on life-long learning. Canadian Medical Association Journal 148: 969–976

Shortridge-Baggett L M, van der Bijl J, Belien M 1994 Utrecht nursing research interest group: development and evaluation. In: Workgroup of European nurse researchers. The contribution of nursing research: past–present–future. 7th Biennial Conference, Oslo, 3–6 July

Skeggs B 1994 Situating the production of feminist ethnography. In: Maynard M, Purvis J (eds) Researching women's lives. Taylor & Francis, London, pp 72–92

Skeggs B 1997 Formations of class and gender: becoming respectable. Sage, London

Smith J P 1979 Is the nursing profession really research based? Journal of Advanced Nursing. 4: 319–325

Smith R 1996 What clinical information do doctors need? British Medical Journal 313: 1062–1068

Social Science Citation Index 1996. Journal citation reports. Institute for Scientific Information, Uxbridge

Soumerai S B 1995 Using research information to promote behavioural change. Proceedings of international conference: Scientific Basis of Health Services, London, 2–4 October, p 28

Spence-Lazinger H K, Foran S, Jones B, Perkins K, Bovan P 1993 Research utilisation in nursing administration – a graduate learning experience. Journal of Nursing Administration 23(2): 32–35

Spurgeon P, Barwell F 1991 Implementing change in the NHS. Chapman & Hall, London

Stetler C B 1994 Refinement of the Stetler-Marram model for the application of research findings to practice. Nursing Outlook 42: 15–25

Stetler C, Marram G 1976 Evaluating research findings for applicability in practice. Nursing Outlook 24: 559–563

Stocking B 1992 Promoting change in clinical care. Quality Health Care 1: 56–60

Stockwell F 1972 The unpopular patient. Royal College of Nursing, London

Street A F 1992 Inside nursing: a critical ethnography of clinical nursing practice. State University of New York Press, New York

Strong P, Robinson J 1990 The NHS under new management. Open University Press, Milton Keynes

Suitor Scheller M K 1993 A qualitative analysis of the factors in the work environment that influence nurses' use of knowledge gained from CE programs. Journal of Continuing Education 24(3): 114–122

Swanson J M, Albright J, Steirn C, Schaffner A, Costa L 1992 Strategies for teaching nursing research: program efforts for creating a research environment in a clinical setting. Western Journal of Nursing Research 14: 241–245

Tanenbaum S J 1994 Knowing and acting in medical practice: the epistemological politics of outcomes research. Journal of Health Politics, Policy and Law 19(1): 27–44

Thompson J 1987 Critical scholarship: the critique of domination in nursing. Advances in Nursing Sciences 10: 27–38

Thiele J 1984 Placement of research: does it make a difference? Western Journal of Nursing Research 6: 356–358

Tibbles L, Sanford R 1994 The research journal club: a mechanism for research utilisation. Clinical Nurse Specialist 8(1): 23–26

Tierney A J 1994 An analysis of nursing's performance in the 1992 assessment of research in British Universities. Journal of Advanced Nursing 19: 593–602

Titler M G, Kleiber C, Steelman V et al 1994 Infusing research into practice to promote quality care. Nursing Research 43: 307–313

Tomlinson B 1992 Report of the inquiry into London's health service, medical education and research. HMSO, London

Tornquist E M, Funk S G, Champagne M T 1995 Research utilization: reconnecting research and practice. AACN Clinical Issues 6(1): 105–109

Traynor M 1996 A literary approach to managerial discourse after the NHS reforms. Sociology of Health and Illness 18: 315–340

Traynor M, Rafferty A M 1997 The NHS R and D context for nursing research: a working paper. Centre for Policy in Nursing Research, London

Ulrich's International Periodicals Directory 1996. Bowker, New York

United Kingdom Central Council for Nursing, Midwifery and Health Visiting 1986 Project 2000: a new preparation for practice. UKCC, London

United Kingdom Central Council for Nursing, Midwifery and Health Visiting 1992 The code of conduct and scope of professional practice. UKCC, London

United Kingdom Central Council for Nursing, Midwifery and Health Visiting 1993 Registrar's letter. The council's position concerning a period of support and preceptorship: implementation of the post-registration education and practice project proposals. UKCC, London

United Kingdom Central Council for Nursing, Midwifery and Health Visiting 1994 The future of professional practice – the council's standards for education and practice following registration. Final draft working paper. UKCC, London

Valente T W, Rogers E M 1995 The origins and development of the diffusion of innovations paradigm as an example of scientific growth. Science Communication 16(3): 242–273

Vas D 1986 An investigation of the usage of the periodical literature of nursing by staff nurses and nursing administrators. Journal of Continuing Education in Nursing 17(1): 22–26

Vaughan B 1989 Two roles – one job. Nursing Times 85(11): 52

Veeramah V 1995 A study to identify the attitudes and needs of qualified staff concerning the use of research findings in clinical practice within mental health settings. Journal of Advanced Nursing 22: 855–861

Verdeber A, Urden L D 1994 A collaborative community model for nursing research: meeting the agenda for the 1990s. Nursing Connections 7(2): 45–51

Walby S, Greenwell J, Mackay L, Soothill K 1994 Medicine and nursing: professions in a changing health service. Sage, London

Walker C 1986 The newly qualified staff nurse's perception of the transition from student to trained nurse. Unpublished MSc thesis, University of Manchester

Walker J F 1993 Teaching and researching in higher education – how is it possible? Nurse Education Today 13: 1–2

Walker J M, Hall S, Thomas M 1995 The experience of labour: a perspective from those receiving care in a midwife-led unit. Midwifery 11: 120–129

Walsh M, Ford P 1989 Nursing rituals: research and rational actions. Heinemann, Oxford

Warmuth J F 1987 In search of the impact of continuing education. Journal of Continuing Education in Nursing 18(1): 4–7

Warner M 1994 Managing monsters: six myths of our time. Vintage, London

White J H 1984 The relationship of clinical practice and research. Journal of Advanced Nursing 9: 181–187

White J M, Leske J S, Pearcy J M 1995 Models and processes of research utilisation. Nursing Clinics of North America 30(3): 409–420

Williams K, Roe B H 1995 Using a handbook to improve nurses' continence care. Nursing Standard 10(8): 39–42

Wilson D 1992 Paradigms and nursing management, analysis of the current organisational structure in a large hospital. Healthcare Management Forum 5: 4–9

Wilson-Barnett J 1997 Evidence for nursing practice – an overview. NT Research Symposium for Evidence-Based Nursing, Manchester. NT Research 2(6): 12–14

Wilson-Barnett J, Corner J, DeCarle B 1990 Integrating nursing research and practice: the role of researcher as teacher. Journal of Advanced Nursing 15: 621–625

Wilson-Barnett J, Butterworth T, White E, Twinn S, Davies S, Riley L 1995 Clinical support and the Project 2000 nursing student: factors influencing this process. Journal of Advanced Nursing 21: 1152–1158

Wilson-Thomas L 1995 Applying critical social theory in nursing education to bridge the gap between theory, research and practice. Journal of Advanced Nursing 1(3): 568–575

Witz A 1992 Professions and patriarchy. Routledge, London

Woolf S H, Battista R N, Anderson G M, Logan A G, Wang E and the Canadian Taskforce on the Periodic Health Examination 1990 Assessing the clinical effectiveness of preventative manoeuvres: analytic principles and systematic methods in reviewing evidence and developing clinical practice recommendations. Journal of Clinical Epidemiology 43: 891–905

Wright S 1997 Perceptions of barriers to implementing research. Nursing Standard 11(19): 34–37

Wright A, Brown P, Sloman R 1996 Nurses' perceptions of the value of nursing research for practice. Australian Journal of Advanced Nursing 13(4): 15–18

Wright M E 1995 A case control study of maternal nutrition and neural tube defects in Northern Ireland. Midwifery 11: 146–152

Wright S, Dolan M 1991 Coming down from the ivory tower. Professional Nurse 7(1): 38–41

Wurman R S 1991 Information anxiety. Pan, London

Subject Index

Page numbers in *italic* print refer to boxed material, figures and tables.

Author Index